HEAD TO TOE
MASSAGE

HEAD TO TOE
MASSAGE

NEW TECHNIQUES FOR
HEALTH AND PLEASURE

D. Baloti Lawrence

A Perigee Book

Perigee Books
are published by
The Putnam Publishing Group
200 Madison Avenue
New York, NY 10016

Library of Congress Cataloging-in-Publication Data

Lawrence, D. Baloti.
Head to toe massage : new techniques for health and pleasure /
D. Baloti Lawrence.

p.   cm.
"A Perigee book."
Includes index.
ISBN 0-399-51442-2
1. Massage.   2. Health.   3. Beauty, Personal.   I. Title.
RA780.5.L37   1988   88-2325 CIP
615.8′22—dc19

Photographs by D. Baloti Lawrence and Ebet Roberts
Illustrations by Fred Bush

Printed in the United States of America
2   3   4   5   6   7   8   9   10

Acknowledgments

Thank you: Marilyn Frender, for showing how to touch; Joan, for the light; Shizuto Masunaga, for the classes—they caused a giant leap in my understanding of the powers of touch; the models—Gayle, Teddy, Terri, Rosie, and Emily; and you, the reader—for taking one more step.

For Mrs. Isabel Riggs and Mrs. Mary F. Friday

Contents

Introduction

Massage is not just relaxing on a table and being stroked. It has a much broader and more far-reaching meaning. The art of touch has many benefits. Touching the body can relieve aches and pains. Touching the mind can release negative emotions and replace them with positive, life-sustaining ones. Touching the spirit can uplift. Touching the world can promote world harmony. Everything we do involves touching, so the applications for massage are unlimited.

Knowing exactly where to touch, how to touch, and when to touch is crucial. Beauty massage can give new meaning to age-old methods used to prevent and remove wrinkles. Massage can be used by a mother to soothe her crying baby. It can also be used by the comforting husband to affectionately caress his wife. Massage offers medical practitioners valuable ways to heal patients.

I have included information on emotional well-being, nutrition, and exercise for a most important reason. The body works as a unit. It is a vast system of systems. Each of these systems has its own function, yet all of them interrelate for the well-being of the whole. Take, for example, the enjoyment of sex. There is no doubt that when sex is lovemaking the entire experience is heightened. Not only does the physical body receive a sensation, the emotional and spiritual bodies are also involved. The pleasure is tripled! In anything we do, having a healthy body and optimally functioning mind will make for a more rewarding experience. And since massage affects the body in many of the same ways that nutrition and exercise do, I discuss all three in this book, hoping that you will unite them for the common cause of looking good and feeling good.

The massage techniques offered in this book offer a bridge between the natural health movement and scientific fitness movements. You might say these are natural techniques with a scientific basis. Many of the techniques can be practiced at home, without help or any expensive aids. All you need is your hands. While the power of being touched by someone is unparalleled and usually most effective, the power of touching yourself is also exhilarating. For this reason, I've included specific self-massage techniques. Getting in touch with yourself doesn't only mean *talking* about your concerns. It literally means having the ability to *feel* yourself, to rediscover yourself, and to love yourself.

I've devoted a great deal of attention in this book to how massage can be useful in a beauty regimen. Some say beauty is a reflection of the inner self. Others say good skin care, along with glamorous cosmetics, is the answer. True beauty requires both. Massage is gaining momentum as a valid and practical method of enhancing beauty from both inside and outside. Proper massage can so reduce facial tension that a person can literally look years younger. That's where massage works on the inner aspect of beauty. But the effect of massage on the circulation and muscle tone can have just as direct an impact on an outwardly beautiful appearance as makeup or even surgery. True beauty reflects physical, mental, social, and spiritual well-being. The ancient art of massage can be beneficial in all of these ways.

Massage will help to improve your health and highlight your personal beauty. It will certainly bring you countless hours of pleasure. So, through this work, I invite you into the world of health, beauty, and pleasure!

1

What to Do to Do It Right

There are several methods of applying massage techniques. How you touch is as important as where you touch. Your intentions, coupled with the correct stroke, knead, or gentle push, will enhance the benefits of massage. By intentions I mean how you feel about what you are doing. Your hands transmit your deeper feelings: If you are feeling melancholy, your touch will reflect it. If you are feeling upset, tense, or angry, these emotions may be transmitted through touch. On the other hand, a relaxed, giving attitude will result in a pleasant, effective touch.

Put another way, the higher the quality of your intentions, the higher the quality of your massage. So when performing any of the techniques in this book, relax, care, and place yourself in a "giving" frame of mind. You will see that this is as important as the techniques themselves.

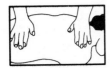

BASIC TECHNIQUES

Effleurage is the French word for stroking. It is a good technique for beginning and ending a massage, or a particular area of bodywork. It is executed by sliding the hands evenly over the body surface with long gliding strokes. The strokes begin lightly, gradually increase in pressure, and taper off at the end.

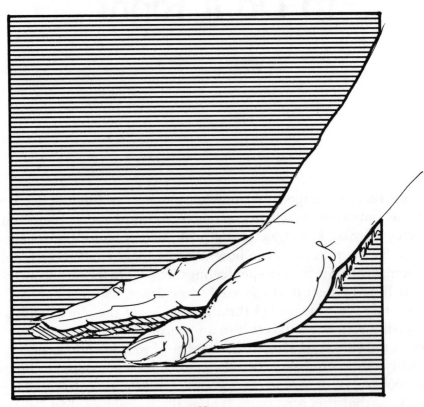

Effleurage.

Petrissage is the French word for kneading. It is a rhythmic lifting, squeezing, pressing, and rolling stroke performed with the hands either stationary or traveling the length of a muscle. The pressure can be increased or decreased, depending on the tone of the muscles and the penetration desired. Both hands may be used alternately to grasp, lift, and gently squeeze the muscles.

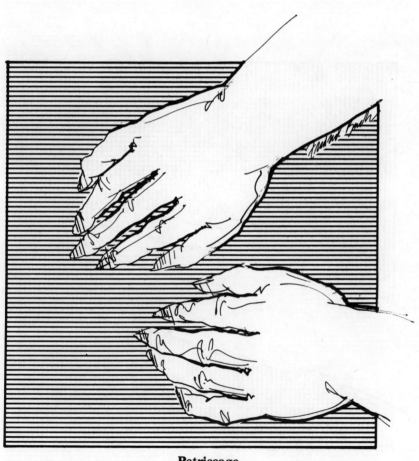

Petrissage.

Friction is performed with the thumb, fingertips, palm, or heel of the hand. It consists of small circular movements varying in pressure. Stiff joints respond well to this technique. Both hands are always kept in contact with the body.

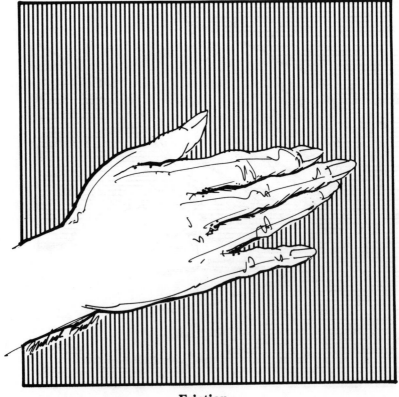

Friction.

Tapotement means percussion in French. It is performed using short, rapid, constantly moving strokes. They may resemble soft karate chops or pitty-pat-like up-and-down movements using the palms or sides of the hands.

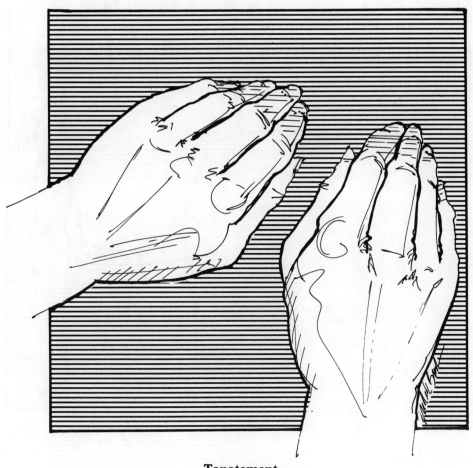

Tapotement.

Range of Motion is a technique used to rotate a body part in a circular movement. First, grasp the joint above and below the joint, gently rock and shake it back and forth, then up and down. Next, rotate the joint in small circles. As resistance decreases, rotate in larger circles.

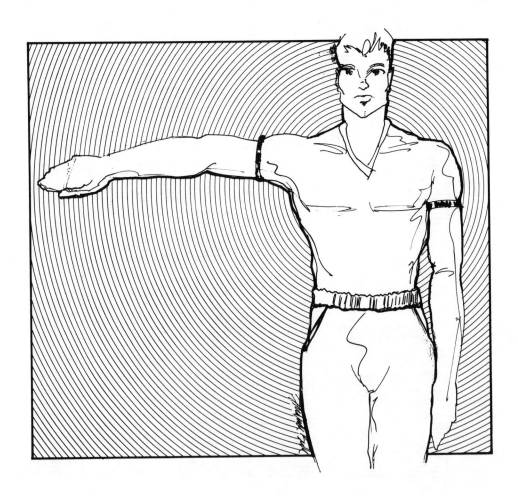

Range of Motion.

Pressure-point Touch may include pressure on acupressure points or special beauty points. To activate them, a gentle finger pressure is used, usually the index finger. In easy-to-reach, sensitive spots, use a light index pressure (some of the points can be extremely sensitive to touch). On deeper or less sensitive spots, use heavier pressure.

Place the finger in the area where you believe the point to be. When you are on it, you or the person may feel a slight tingling or warming sensation. You will know when you reach it simply because it feels like the "right" place to be. If you are not on the point exactly, but you feel heat, or sensations, stay right there; chances are that is a better spot anyway! Apply pressure for anywhere from 3 to 15 seconds.

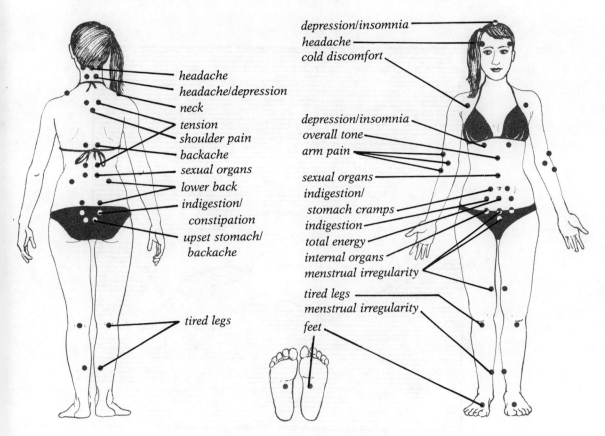

Important pressure points.

Dancing Fingers is a movement designed to release tension from an area while it also stimulates it pleasurably. Lightly tap and move the fingers over the forehead, chest, or face.

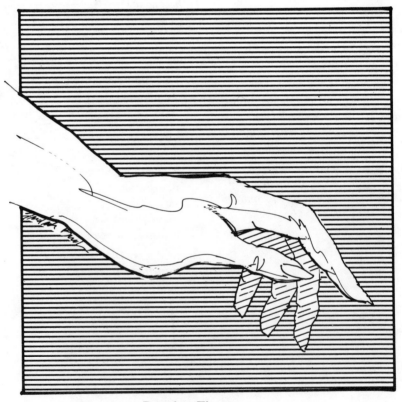

Dancing Fingers.

The Benefits of Massage

1. Mechanical cleanser (increases the interchange of tissue fluids emptied into the capillaries and lymphatic system)
2. Improves circulation
3. Brings about a state of general relaxation
4. Adds to overall well-being
5. Relieves muscle spasms
6. Improves muscle tone
7. Redirects negative energy
8. Produces an alpha state in which body and mind are totally relaxed
9. Promotes good digestion
10. Relieves head, neck, and backache
11. Reduces cellulite and varicose veins
12. Helps in sports injuries
13. Helps release negative and pent-up emotions
14. Helps firm and soften skin
15. Helps remove toxins from skin
16. Helps relieve tensions
17. Gives a glowing appearance to skin
18. Helps break down fatty tissue
19. Stretches tight muscles
20. Helps open and clear sinuses
21. Increases joint mobility
22. Relieves tired and sore muscles
23. Improves self-esteem
24. Dilates blood vessels
25. Increases nutrient distribution in the body
26. Improves condition of arthritic joints
27. Useful in bursitis, tendonitis
28. Helps stimulate cell activity and hair growth
29. Helps prevent wrinkles
30. Helps relieve menstrual cramps

IT FEELS GOOD!!!

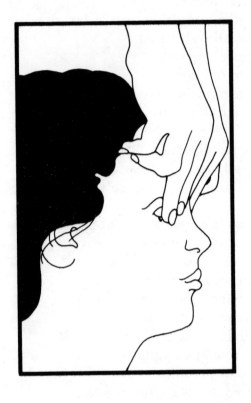

2
Attitudes About Touch

When you touch, make sure that your head and heart are in the right place. Touching is caring. Touching is loving. Touching is feeling. Everyone has the ability to touch. Everyone has feelings.

Touching can be a very personal matter. Each of us may touch the same object and feel very different sensations. Touch is a two-way process: Feeling is sent and feeling is received. If there is something troubling you and you touch someone else, he or she may immediately feel it. On the other hand, when you are feeling great your positive emotion will also be transferred through your touch.

Don't be afraid to touch. Try for a moment to touch yourself. Feel parts of your body you have not touched in a while. Feel the texture of your hair. Touch your face with your fingertips. Touch your eyebrow with the tip of your pinkie. Explore.

Touching is an art, whether it is the sensual caress of lovers or the firm stroke of a sports massage, whether it is the calming tummy rock from a mother to her restless baby or the grasping of a congratulatory handshake. Hugging is another form of touching, a very healthy one. A touch can be just what the doctor ordered!

Touching can have several characteristics: It can be a squeeze, or it can be a grasp, or it can be a cling. It can be light, or it can be firm. It can be a grip or it can be a tap, a punch, a stroke, or a pull. The form of touch is not as important as the intention. The intention is a reflection of the inner feelings. Somehow I cannot help but feel that all things truly begin within and are simply magnified and exhibited in the physical world. Keep in mind that a good touch always starts from *within*.

For several reasons, this simple action—touching—provides hours of pleasure. But we often hold back from letting ourselves express our deeper and truer feelings. We often forget to give that healing, loving touch.

Touching provides a way of emphasizing some of our innermost feelings. When words will not or cannot express something, surrender to the feeling of a warm hug. Watch the barriers and tensions melt away. On a much wider level, what if the men and women who decide issues of war or world peace started each meeting with a happy laugh and a warm hug? Surely it would help ease the anxiety and start things off on a healthy, positive note, allowing dialogue and discussion to be intelligent and free of tension.

Touch can be expanded to include all forms of communication. What about words, for instance? Can we provide pleasure and good health with words? Do words have a therapeutic effect on the body? Negative, angry, jealous, or vengeful words arouse low self-esteem, anxiety, and tense muscles. On the other hand, the right words can relax tense muscles and afford the listener much glowing pleasure. Touching with positive, joyful, or complimentary words is felt as a health-supporting sensation.

Test yourself. Look into the mirror and say "I hate you." Look into it again and say "I love you." You'll feel the difference. Gentle words can be an important part of a good massage.

At a time when heavy emphasis is being placed on relationships, one gets the feeling that cuddling and hugging will become more a part of our world. And so they should, because they will only help us get closer to the true source of health and pleasure deep within our souls. Knowing yourself and feeling good about yourself presents a certain aura. This is not to say everyone does not have their ups and downs; life is, after all, a struggle we must face each day. It does mean, however, that in living each day we can have more control over our lives. Why not choose happiness over worry? Why not a vibrant life of activity over a critical, sedentary one? Why not pleasure over pain?

In this simple concept of touch, a whole world of discovery awaits us, about ourselves and the world we live in. Yet many people find it difficult to touch or hug. Hugging is not just for babies and children. Everyone needs more of it. Just keep in mind that it's okay to show your inner feelings sometimes.

This is one of the reasons that the right massage can be so wonderful. Often it's a godsend for people who, for one reason or another, are afraid to be touched or find it difficult to touch others. If the touch is in the right place and offered with the right sensitivity and intention behind it, even the most resistant person will experience a marvelous sensation. As muscle after muscle relaxes and breathing reaches a harmonious flow, the entire body is calmed.

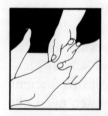

THE RIGHT TOUCH

Everyone can have a special touch; everyone can bring joy to themselves and to others through this "special touch." It is warm, it is in the right place, and it has the right intentions.

How does one perform this kind of touch? Here are some general rules that can be helpful:

- Locate in your own mind what you will be touching yourself or the other person with. Will you be using one finger, four fingers, your palm, the side of your hand?
- Knowing where to touch is as important as how you touch. It can mean the difference between pleasure and pain. So, begin by visualizing the area and just touch it, without moving.
- Take a deep breath, slowly inhaling and even more slowly exhaling. Gradually begin your stroke or technique.

The softer the better; that way it lasts longer. Being gentle can be both calming and stimulating. Take time in your touch. Allow yourself to feel; don't rush it. A moment of real pleasure is good both to you and for you. This method works every time for touching yourself or others.

You can probably feel your way to happiness if you really try. As the saying goes, "Get in touch with yourself." You'll be a lot better for it. Treating yourself well and feeling sensual is both healthy and pleasurable. It is both good *to* you and good *for* you.

The right touch can provide the right feelings. Touching and feeling don't have to be strangers in our relationships with ourselves or with others who may be close to us. Love touches deeper than any feeling imaginable. Loving is a pleasurable experience, as is being loved. When we learn more about touching we may in fact be learning how to love more. Feeling the touch of love is the ultimate good feeling.

Massage, which is a healing art, is also extremely sensual. It necessarily involves touching. While touching need not be sexual at all in performing massage, massage done purely for the sake of sexual pleasure—though not the subject of this book—is a high form of this ancient art. But in doing head-to-toe massage, remember that a touch need not be sexual to be sensual. Enjoy every sensuous touch to the fullest.

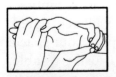

HARD OR SOFT?

Don't worry about how much pressure to apply. If you are massaging yourself, remember that it doesn't have to hurt to be good for you. Pleasure in life, and pleasure in all things, is all right to have for oneself. Some people have the mistaken idea that massage must be painful to be effective. In my experience, the better it feels, the more effective it will be. This is so with anything we do. The better it is enjoyed, the better it is for us.

Therefore, the lighter approach is better. Approach the body as the temple of miracles it actually is. Caress it, examine it, touch it with warm, open, and loving hands.

By taking this approach, you can be assured that massage is already working. The body both feels and appreciates the tender care. Begin with light pressure, and gradually apply more pressure. Continue to increase the pressure as the person receiving offers less resistance and as your touch becomes more in tune with the person's bodily reactions.

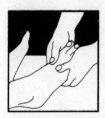

HELPFUL HINTS

Before starting the massage, rub your hands together until you feel a warming sensation. Then gently place the hands on the face as your first contact. Just relax, take a deep breath. Now begin.

Environment is important. Make sure there are no interruptions once the session begins. The space should be warm and well ventilated. For variety, select your favorite music and colors to prepare your space. Of course, any other creative ideas are always a plus. If using a table, make sure it is secure and comfortable. Keep in mind that massage lowers blood pressure and body temperature. Since the person may feel cold after the session, wrap them in a sheet or covering of some type. After the session shake your hands and rinse them in cold water. This will help the circulation in your hand and rid it of any excess energy from the session. Often, at the end of a session, the giver can feel as delightful as the receiver. Massage works that way. It is truly a two-way process.

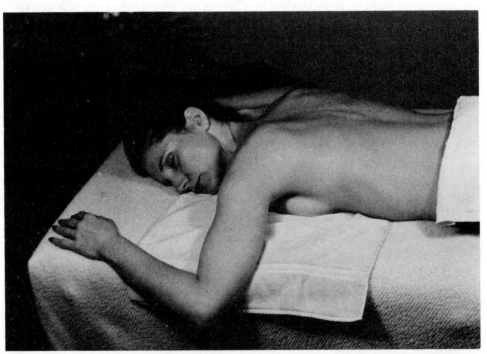

After a session, it is most beneficial to lie still for a while to soak in the relaxed afterglow.

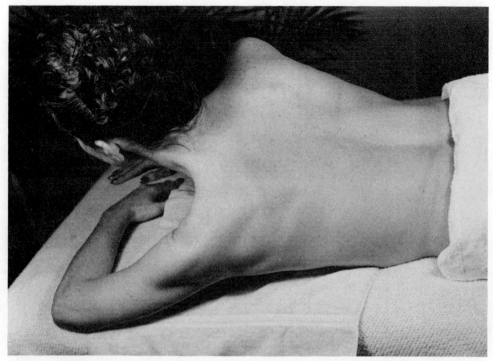

When getting up, do so slowly to allow the body a chance to balance itself.

SELF TECHNIQUE: The massage technique you can use on yourself.
EXERCISE: A specific exercise that works along with the technique, to be done daily.
ESTHETIC TECHNIQUE: A technique used by massage practitioners.
BEAUTY POINTS: Special points to which pressure is applied.

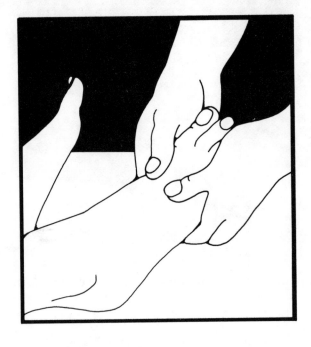

3

The Anatomy of Energy Systems

All that *is* cannot be seen by the naked eye. *Qi* or *chi* is a basic concept of Eastern thought. Defined as the life force, *qi* energy circulates throughout the body in specific directions. *Qi* in the human body is supported by eating, breathing, exercise, and massage. It is the body's vital energy. Imbalance in this vital energy is a cause for physical, social, or emotional imbalance, and many of the changes in life are manifested in this energy system. An ancient Chinese philosopher wrote: "That which was born from the beginning in heaven is Qi, on earth it becomes visible as form. Qi and form interact, giving birth to the myriad of things."

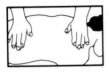

YIN AND YANG

In Oriental theory, there is a constant struggle in the human body between opposing and unifying forces: hot vs. cold, wet vs. dry, up vs. down, anger vs. love, etc. Good health is affected by these forces. The two polar forces in which universal energy is manifested are known as yin and yang. Yin has female properties, and yang has male properties, although yin has some male traits, while yang has some female properties. When working together, they comprise a complete entity. Just as these two forces are in constant conflict, they are in constant harmony. When the two are in harmony, there is ultimate health and beauty. When either principle is in excess, there may be an imbalance. It is a constant balancing of these two forces and the principles they represent that brings about a pleasurable and healthy existence.

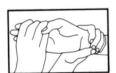

THE FIVE-ELEMENT THEORY

This concept is not unique or mystical. It is a traditional mode of thinking that postulates that the atmosphere in which we live controls our bodies to some extent. It holds that our bodies are composed of these very same elements. Therefore, it is from their existence that our existence derives. So it is thought that by understanding the ways and properties of these elements, we can better understand ourselves. Each element and its properties has a certain influence over our sense organs, body parts, and internal organs. Thus, in Oriental philosophy, man, woman, and nature share many qualities.

As you can see on page 36, each element affects a certain organ. Each organ is defined as either yin (passive) or yang (active). In addition, each organ has a pair. When there is imbalance in one organ the associated organ may also have an imbalance.

Energy pathways carry the *qi*. These pathways, called meridians, are related to element theory in that the body elements are vehicles for the movement of *qi*. When energy is flowing properly in the organs, the result is total harmony, or "beauty of the highest order, both inside and out."

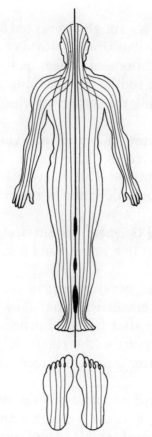

The body's energy meridians, which circulate the vital quality known as *qi*.

Some meridians start at the feet and run the length of the body to the face and head. You might say that the meridians are a form of circulatory system that carries the precious vital energy known as *qi*, instead of moving blood or food. Along the pathways, there are various points the size of a pin head that have a great effect on the flow of energy when pressed, rubbed, or heated. These points are called *tsubos (su bose)*. *Tsubos* are beginning and ending points for energy flows. To increase energy in a certain part of the body one can locate the *tsubos* or energy connections that relate to that point. In each section of this book we give specific energy points for the part of the body being discussed and for specific applications, including weight loss and the prevention and reduction of wrinkles.

Oriental philosophy is strongly connected to the balance that occurs in nature and in our relationship to natural conditions. Food can build energy *(qi)*, weather conditions can affect *qi*, exercise can strengthen or deplete *qi*, massage can soothe *qi*. Anything that has a positive and nourishing effect will bring the total body closer to the goal of physical and mental harmony.

Since the Oriental view of health involves harmony between man and the universe, the activities, the behavior, and the qualities of man and nature are seen as similar. This relationship between man and nature can help us to understand some of the whys, hows, and whats of our condition.

The elements in the Oriental system are wood, fire, earth, metal, and water. Each can exist in a helpful and complementary relationship with the others.

The relationship and development of the elements has a certain pattern and there is a certain way that they work together. Fire, for example, is fed by wood. After fire has burned itself out, the ashes feed the earth. Metals develop from the earth. When metals are dissolved they form liquids, the water from which feeds the trees, thus completing the cycle back to wood.

This cyclical relationship in nature is also associated with the human experience. Each of the elements has a human emotional and physical relationship: Earth represents stability and substance, fertility, etc. Fire, on the other hand, represents energy, movement, and dynamics. As we interact with our environment, the forces of nature are at work, assuming an important role in shaping our lives. The Oriental philosophy of health stresses the relationship between humankind and nature, as they rely upon, influence, and affect each other day to day.

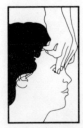

BODY AURAS AND CHAKRAS

Energy is not visible to the naked eye, but that does not mean that it does not exist. Likewise, the aura, a system composed of energy that usually emanates outside of our bodies, cannot usually be seen. It is a luminous, colored form of light that surrounds the body. In many ancient Greek and Egyptian paintings this body of surrounding light was depicted in the form of halos in pictures of angels, or as a haze of light around great heroes.

Constantly in motion, auras react to the condition of the internal body and the environment. If your body is in harmony and health, your aura will glow brightly. Your light will shine, your presence will be felt, your energy will be giving off its impression, and your total being will be one of great beauty. The aura both sends and receives energy. Negative thoughts that penetrate it may diminish it. Positive thoughts, quality food, and nourishing social interaction will enhance it. The aura can extend up to six or seven feet from the body.

Like the *tsubos*, the eight chakras are special energy points along the aura that can be used in massage. These energy points each has a certain influence. Located in a horizontal line from the reproductive organs to the top of the head, they receive and distribute energy between

Table of Elements, Qualities, and Organs

CHAKRA	ROOT	HARA	SOLAR PLEXUS	HEART	THROAT	BROW	CROWN
GLAND	ADRENAL	GONADS	PANCREAS	THYMUS	THYROID	PITUITARY	ALL GLANDS
PHYSICAL PART	LEGS FEET GENITALS COCCYX KIDNEYS ANUS	PELVIS GENITAL/REPRODUCTIVE BELLY SACRUM LUMBAR	STOMACH GALL BLADDER LIVER DIAPHRAGM NERVOUS SYSTEM	HEART LOWER LUNGS CHEST BREASTS THORACIC CIRCULATORY SYSTEM	ARMS HANDS THROAT MOUTH LUNGS CERVICAL RESPIRATORY SYSTEM	FOREHEAD EAR LOBE NOSE EYE BASE OF SKULL MEDULLA NERVOUS SYSTEM	HEAD BRAIN EARS SPINE
BEHAVIOR	PHYSICAL WILL TO BE; PRIMAL SEXUAL SURVIVAL	VITALITY MOVEMENT SEXUAL EXPRESSION GROUNDING	RAW EMOTION ENERGY DESIRE PERSONAL POWER	LOVE COMPASSION SERVICE TO HUMANITY	SELF-EXPRESSION CREATIVITY CLAIRAUDIENCE	INTUITION INTELLECT CLAIRVOYANCE	SPIRITUALITY PASSION HUMANITY EVOLUTION PROGRESS

the physical body and the emotional body. Balance among the chakras is important, just as balance in all of our organs is important. The chart on the opposite page shows the interconnection of the chakras and the parts of the body.

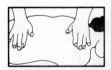

THE BODY-ENERGY CONNECTION

Energy, our physical bodies, and our emotional bodies are infinitely interrelated. Vitality is the sum total of their smooth operation. Vitality occurs when there is an optimal flow of energy through the entire system. This flow best occurs when there is harmony, peace of mind, and physical health.

All things have an energy. Talk to botanists, and they will speak of the energy of plants; speak with physicians, and they will speak of the energy of heart rates and blood pressure; listen to scientists, and they will speak of solar energy.

All living things are in movement, growth, change, and refinement. With each change, there is a change of energy; with each change in energy, there is a new experience. Each movement sends off a vibration. Often, we can read these vibrations in others; perhaps how they are feeling, and in many cases what they are thinking. Since thoughts are living things, they too have vibrations. You've heard the expression, "Be careful what you wish for, it might come true." Thoughts are a movement of the mind. They have to do with wishes, feelings, and desires. Talking is merely a physical, oral interpretation of those thoughts.

Energy affects our lives in everything we do, eat, or experience. Positive energies usually indicate a happier, healthier life. Here are some helpful tips to keep positive energy working for you:

- Vegetables and fruits have more positive energy than meats. Fresh, crisp fruits and vegetables have more positive energy than wilted ones.
- Fresh air increases the body's vitality while smoke-filled or polluted air drains vitality and ages the body prematurely.
- Considerate, kind, or helpful gestures have more energy than harsh, mean, anxiety-prone gestures.
- Too much stress destroys valuable energy, while a little stress may help to increase it.
- Colors affect our energy—while red excites the body, violet relaxes it.
- Thoughts, feelings, attitudes, and relationships all affect our energy.
- Excess energy with no direction may be stressful.
- The average human uses only 25 percent of his or her true energy potential.
- Love, desire, hope, faith, and inner confidence all have high vibratory waves, while despair, anger, jealousy, and fear have low vibrational frequency.
- Herbs, flowers, and water have high vibrations.
- Things with high vibrational qualities are healthy and vital, producing a state of total harmony.
- Things with low vibrational qualities deplete valuable energy.
- The entire world is realizing a faster pace and greater demand of personal energy.

Staying in stride and being healthy have a lot in common. They both require energy—the right kind of energy. While massage relaxes the entire body, it also energizes it; recharges its low batteries; rejuvenates its cells; clears out its clogged energy channels. As tensions are relieved, oxygen is exchanged and invigorating actions start occurring. Immediately after a massage, the body is usually heavy and somewhat sluggish. Sometime later, however, it feels invigorated, fresh, and vital.

Energy is in all things; it ties together in a giant reservoir of human life, with my energy affecting the next person, and that person's energy affecting the life of the next, and on and on. We are all connected by a vast network of physical, emotional, and spiritual energies. The moment there is breath, there is life. And life can be as we want it to be. We can invite positive vibrations into our lives or we can invite negative vibrations. The choice is ours.

The fragrance of a red rose, the soothing stroking of a tired muscle, or the receiving of a timely promotion all produce a certain kind of energy. Can you guess what it is? It's not hard. Just ask yourself, How does it make me feel? Is it good for me or not? Does it create vitality in my life or does it dissipate it? Most of all, does it make me a happier, healthier person?

People have differing needs. But one thing is for sure: There is nothing wrong with fulfilling our needs, pampering ourselves a bit, and increasing our own energy and vitality by attracting positive energy and avoiding, wherever possible, the influence of negative energy.

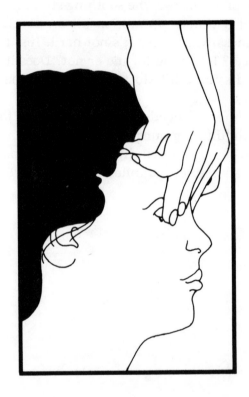

4
Heads Up! Massaging the Head

At the very top of the body is one of its most sensitive parts: the head. It houses that delicate element known as the brain, which requires more oxygen than other parts of the body. When the brain doesn't get all it needs, muscles tighten and become tense. When muscles in the head tighten, the facial muscles also tighten; thus tension in the head causes premature wrinkling in the face. If the head muscles relax or release, facial muscles will also. Try for a moment to tighten the sides of your head by squeezing both sides toward the center of your head. Feel the place where your face expresses a corresponding tightness.

When blood vessels constrict, the result is head tension, which, if left unrelieved, will result in a headache. There are various types of headaches, among them the classic and migraine headaches. While they have different causes, and may occur in different parts of the head, all are uncomfortable and painful.

Some Causes of Headaches

caffeine (coffee, chocolate, certain teas)
dairy products (for some individuals)
smoking
alcohol
stress and anxiety
worry
lack of fresh air
additives (nitrites, red dye, etc.)
excessive salt intake
loud noises
lack of exercise
tense neck and shoulder muscles

THE IMPORTANCE OF HEAD MASSAGE

Since the ability to feel sensations is a brain function, those who have stress or discomfort in the head cannot possibly feel the full spectrum of pleasures in life. Sensations are perceived and sent to various parts of the body from the head. So, you might say a tension-free head frees the rest of the body to experience all the pleasures of life.

Along with massage, a total approach—talking out your problems, letting go of worry, and a better diet—will bring long-lasting effects and will help alleviate head tension. The following self techniques, however, will in most cases provide immediate but temporary relief.

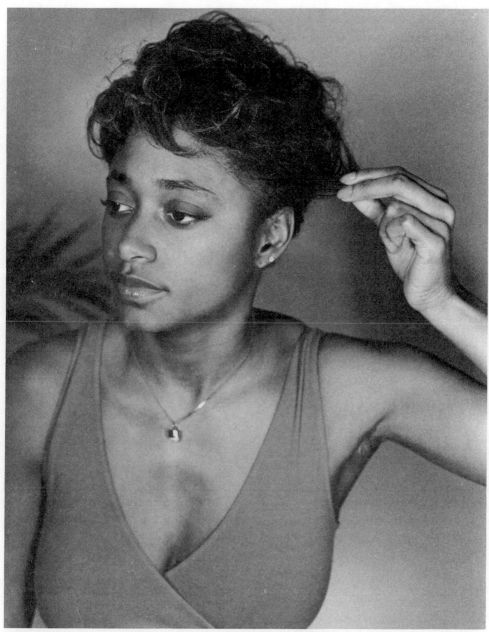

A technique to stimulate the scalp and draw out the tension: Gently pull the hair and rotate it around and around. Repeat this over the entire head.

1. Beginning at the base of the neck on both sides of the head, use an open hand to stroke up to the top of the head.

2. Gently shake your head, first from side to side, then up and down.

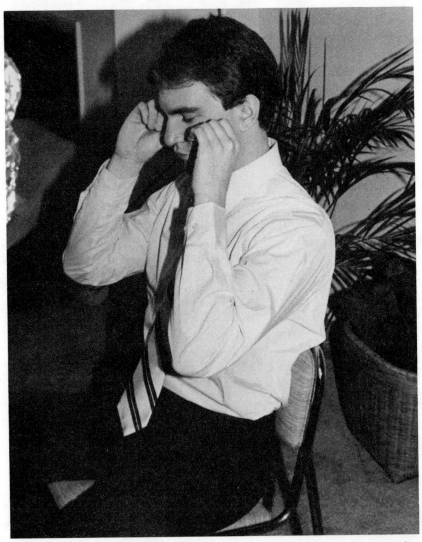

Relieving nagging head tension at work: Apply pressure to the cheek on both sides.

The next series of techniques for relieving head tension can be done on yourself as well as on others.

1. Inhale and visualize the area where the pain or tension exists. As you exhale, envision a stream of water flowing from your head and out with the breath. Repeat this three times, each time visualizing more and more tension as it flows out.

If possible, just sit quietly for about fifteen minutes. Turn off the lights, the radio, TV, and telephone. Lean back and close your eyes. Become aware of your breathing.

2. Place the palms on the temples. With a slow, pulsating motion, squeeze gently, hold for a few counts, and release. Repeat for about a minute or two. Next, move both hands half the distance to the back of the head and repeat. Finally, squeeze gently at the very back of the head.

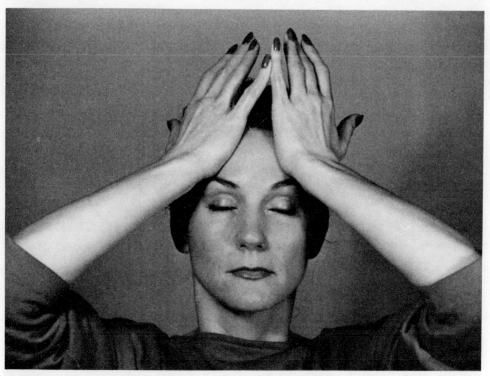

Massaging the temples using the palms of the hands.

3. With the tips of the hands, roam lightly around the entire head in a "scratching" motion. This is both an effective and pleasurable technique.

4. Locate the center top of the head. Draw an imaginary straight line from there to the top of both ears. Now draw another imaginary line from the center of the eyebrows to that line. Find the place where the two points meet. Immediately around this area you will feel a slight indentation. Apply pressure to this point using your middle finger. Press lightly and hold for about fifteen seconds. Repeat four or five times.

5. Rotate the neck. (Neck rotations help release tension from over-stressed neck and shoulder muscles, which may cause head tension.) Rotate the entire head, using the neck as the axis. Rotate clockwise three or four times, then counterclockwise. Try rotating in slow, small circles first, then gradually increasing to slow, large circles. Try to breathe out

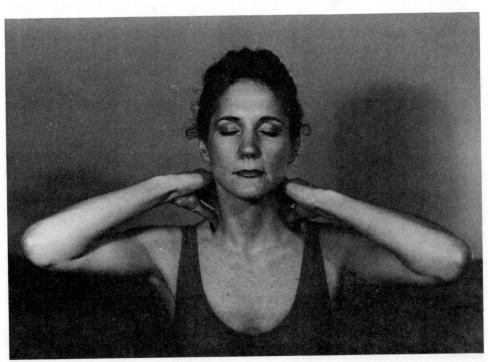

Kneading the neck.

the tension through coordinated inhalations and exhalations.

6. Try the Dancing Fingers technique. Lightly tap the entire head area, using only the tips of all ten fingertips in a "dancing" (tapping) motion.

7. Knead the neck. Beginning at the base of the skull, on the back of the head, knead the large muscle located on either side of the spine. Work your way to the base of the neck, near the large bone. Knead for three or four minutes.

8. Massage the special headache point in the neck. Apply gentle pressure to the point as you follow the general guidelines for applying pressure. Hold the pressure for fifteen or twenty seconds. Repeat three times. This point is located on the center of the back of the neck. You will find it midway between the seventh cervical vertebra (the large bone that protrudes when you drop your head) and the base of the skull.

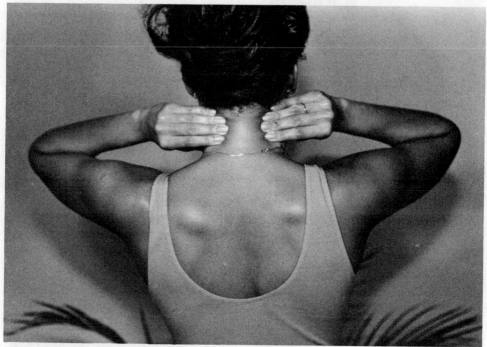

Massaging the special headache point in the neck, which lies between the base of the skull and the last vertebra.

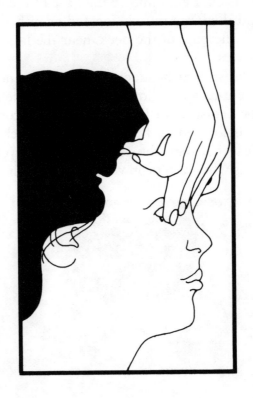

5

Esthetic Massage
for the Face

Esthetic massage follows the natural contours of the muscles. And since facial muscles connect the movements and structure of the face, to some extent they determine the way we look. If we smile broadly, the sides near the nose develop a line. Over time, the line gets heavier and heavier. If we frown, we may drop the eyebrows, and eventually the brows will sag. If we worry excessively, horizontal lines may increase in the forehead area.

Toning all the facial muscles relieves them of tension and helps increase circulation in the surface skin. Facial massage is a means of preventing, diminishing, and in some cases even eliminating unwanted lines and wrinkles. Most assuredly, it will help bring that special individual beauty to your skin. And—when used in conjunction with proper nutrition, exercise, visualization, and a positive attitude—it will take years off your face.

Ultimately, facial beauty is the result of two factors: happiness, which radiates from within, creating a vibrant glow on the outside; and physical health, which results from proper nutrition, exercise, and emotional well-being. Of course, well-chosen cosmetics, clothes, and jewelry can help, but they can only highlight what is already there. A warm personality, confidence, a sense of security, and the ability to enjoy life are traits of the most "beautiful" people I have ever met.

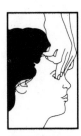

SMILE AND THE WORLD SMILES WITH YOU

Facial massage will improve your skin by increasing circulation, giving you a glowing complexion. Underutilized facial muscles can benefit from the stimulation produced by massage, and overutilized ones can be soothed by massage. Massage may also prevent, and in some cases, alleviate, unwanted lines. Beneath the skin lie muscles, blood vessels, fat, bones, and connective tissues, all of which are involved with your face's cosmetic appearance.

Muscle and bone give the face its shape. Weak facial muscles will mean sagging cheeks or a jowly jaw. Keep in mind that each movement, each expression, each blush, frown, laugh, or pout is shown in the face. Every muscle in the face has a creative function. Every one is connected in action to another. They work together like a pulley; when one gets longer or stretches, a corresponding one contracts and gets shorter. When one muscle is used over and over, it leaves deep lines. Massage can help correct this imbalanced usage.

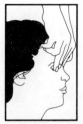

TRY A COMPLEXION BRUSH

Using a complexion brush is one way to treat your face to a pleasurable experience. Complexion brushes designed especially for the contour of the facial structure are best when made from 100% silk bristles. When applying moisturizer, it becomes a self-massage brush. Simply use it after washing your face, following the contour of your face, especially around the jawline, forehead, cheekbone, and neck. In addition to feeling soft and silky, it helps to increase circulation in your face.

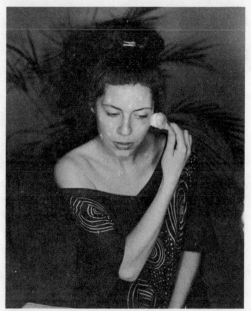

Stroking the face with a silk brush. Stroke wherever there is a bone; simply follow the natural contour of your face, stroking upward wherever possible. Do this with or without moisturizer.

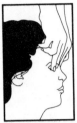

HOW TO GIVE YOURSELF A FACIAL

Treating yourself to a facial can be a wonderful way of pampering your-self. Here's a five-step program. I recommend using natural ingredients whenever possible.

1. *Cleanse*—A milk cleanser or gentle soap will gently wash away makeup while it penetrates deep onto the soft cellular tissues to remove

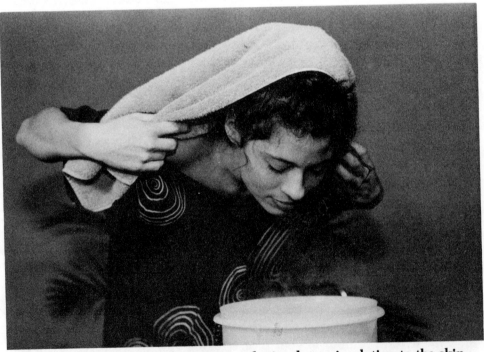

A facial steam bath cleans out pores and stimulates circulation to the skin.

excess dirt and open clogged pores. Gently massage the skin using circular motions. Rinse with warm water, follow with cool water. Your regular cleansing routine should be done every morning and evening.

2. *Steam*—An herbal sauna is a delightful penetrating mist that deep-cleans your pores and stimulates your skin for a healthier complexion. Boil 3 cups of water. Put 1 tablespoon each of camomile, eucalyptus, and peppermint into a bowl and pour the boiling water over it. Cover your head with a towel, creating a "tent." Place your head 10 inches above the bowl to allow the steam to penetrate your face. Rinse your face with warm water, follow with cool water. Oily skin types should use this steaming technique three to four times a week.

3. *Refine*—An exfoliating mask renews, cleanses, and refines your skin, working into the soft cellular tissue to add nourishing enzymes. It removes dead skin cells and leaves a healthy and youthful skin surface. Gently massage a basic cleansing mask into your skin and allow it to dry. Leave it on for 15–20 minutes. Oily skin types should use a mask three times a week; those with dry skin, once a week or as needed.

Here is a recipe for a basic cleansing mask:

4 tablespoons whole oatmeal
3 tablespoons plain yogurt
OPTIONAL: for dry skin, 1 avocado; for normal skin, avocado or peach slices.

Mix all ingredients in a blender until smooth.

4. *Tone*—Toners bond your skin, leaving you with a refreshing feeling. Avoid using toners with alcohol, as it both dries and de-vitaminizes your skin. Several herbs may be used in a basic toner because of their astringent qualities. Other useful ingredients include witch hazel, glycerine, and rose oil or flowers, mixed as follows:

2 ounces glycerine
dash rose oil
4 ounces witch hazel

Apply a basic toner with cotton and gently smooth it over your entire face and throat. Use it daily as an astringent or refresher.

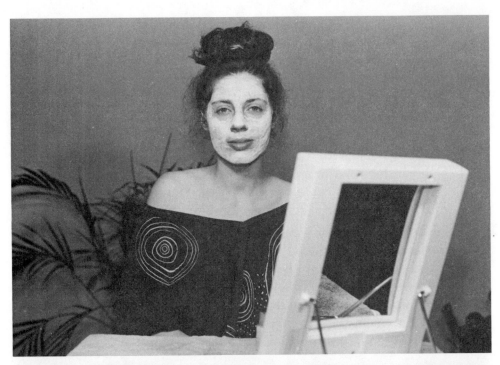

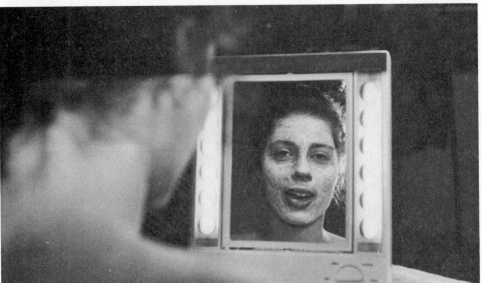

An exfoliating mask can be quite flattering.

5. *Moisturize and Renew*—Using a moisture cream is the final step of your beauty regime, sealing in moisture and renewing soft cellular tissue. This leaves your skin vibrant and healthy. Gently massage the cream into your skin. Use daily or at night.

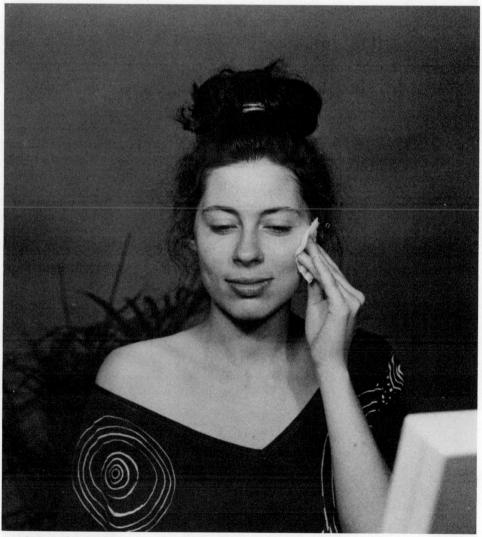

Applying skin toner.

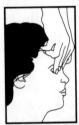

MASSAGING THE FACE

When you are massaging the face, touch it gently, and in a caring way. It is a most sensitive organ. Its parts too are sensitive and in most cases small. They require a very special approach.

Each part of the face has specific techniques or exercises that you may apply.

Eyes

Often, congestion or blocked energy will create a slightly swollen appearance just above the brow. The eyes may not appear open, bubbly, or bright; the brows will droop and appear to cover the eyes. Facial problems that result are crow's-feet, squinting, excessive winking, and puffiness under the eyes.

Self technique: Look up, down, left, and right, moving only your eyes. Look up as though you are trying to see your forehead. Hold your eyebrows up for ten seconds. Massage circles around your eyes.

Esthetic technique: Use round strokes around the eyes. Begin at the brow and work to the top of cheek. Make smaller circles, then larger ones.

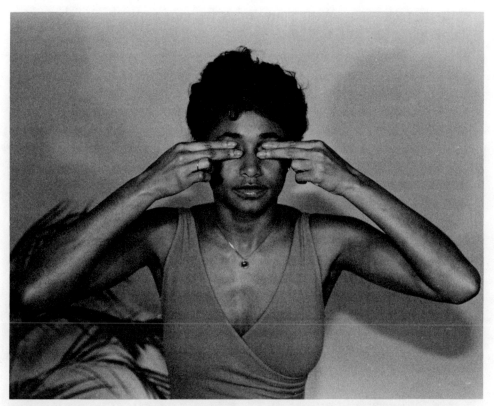

Rejuvenating the eyes. Place the index and middle fingers over closed eyes, applying gentle pressure. Then gently rotate fingers in both directions.

The muscles that raise the upper eyelid can keep them raised if they are tense, giving a "knitted brow" look, or they can, if weak, give the eyelids a saggy look. They terminate in the deep surface of the skin of the upper eyelid. The functional part of this muscle is behind the eye.

Self technique: Place your fingers under the ridge of your eyelids and push the eyebrows up.

Exercise: Open your eyes as wide as possible.

Esthetic technique: With your index finger, locate the forehead's energy center and massage with circular motions.

Beauty point for acupressure: Center of eyebrow. (See diagram of the face's beauty points, page 75.)

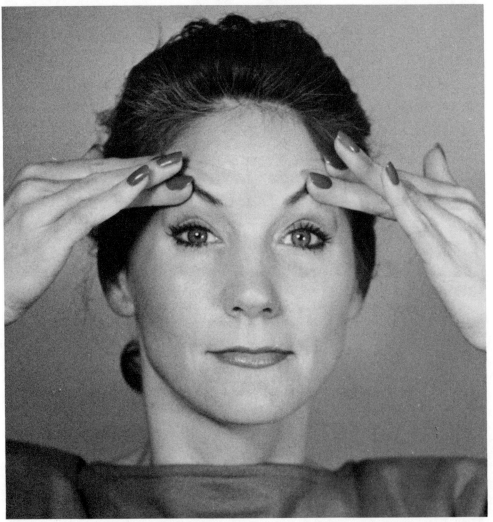

Massaging the eyelid and eyebrow.

Forehead

The corrugator is a small muscle that extends from the middle of the forehead to the middle of the upper eyelid. When it contracts, it wrinkles the forehead and draws the eyebrows inward. Therefore it draws the brows down and to the center, creating so-called worry lines.

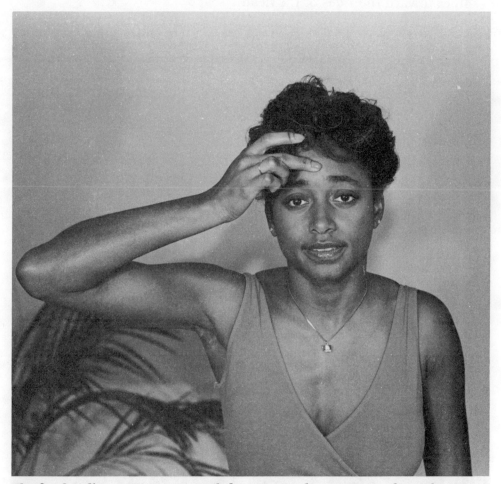

The forehead's energy center. Lightly press on the point just above the center of the eyebrows. Press three times, holding for about ten seconds each time. This helps clear the mind.

Self technique: Hold your eyelids between your fingertips and pull toward the ears on both sides.

Exercise: Gazing straight ahead, look surprised. Open and stretch your entire face. Look to the right ear with your right eye, and to the left ear with your left eye.

Esthetic technique: Using the fingertips, gently stroke the worry lines toward the sides of the head.

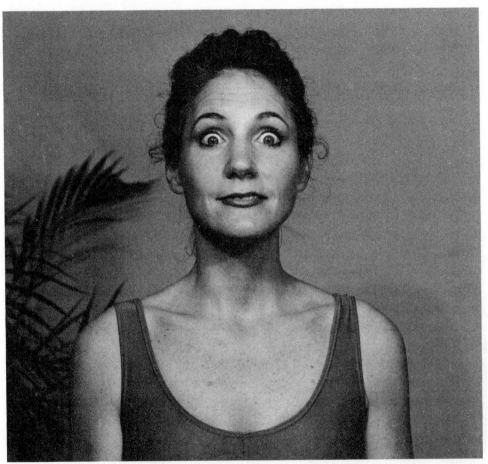

Looking surprised to uplift the entire face and prevent sagging.

Nose

The procerus muscle attaches to the skin of the nose and the skin of the forehead, drawing the brows together. The muscle looks like a pyramid in its structure. It begins at the lower part of the nasal bone and ends between the eybrows. It also controls wrinkles at the bridge of the nose.

Self technique: Stroke the nose as in the esthetic technique.

Exercise: Pull the forehead up from the eyes, at the same time pulling the bottom of the face from the bridge of the nose down.

Esthetic technique: Apply transverse stroking at the top of the nose and transverse stroking along the entire nose.

Beauty point for acupressure: Corner of nostrils.

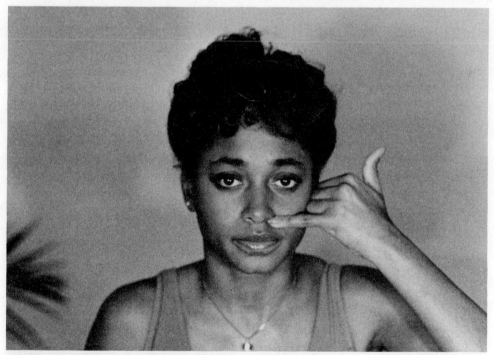

Massaging the beauty points. Place the small finger at the corner of each nostril and hold for about ten seconds.

Mouth

The oral muscles work to open and close the mouth. The circular muscle that surrounds the opening of the mouth helps form the shape of the lips. It ends at the base of the nose; the lower portion ends at the cleft in the chin.

Self technique: Pull your lips and hold the corners.

Exercise: Spread your lips wide to the side, in a wide grin. Then pucker them.

Esthetic technique: Using the fingertips, massage clockwise at least six times, then massage counterclockwise an equal number of times.

Beauty point for acupressure: Corner of lips.

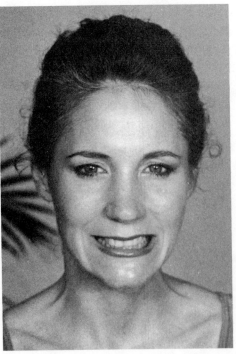 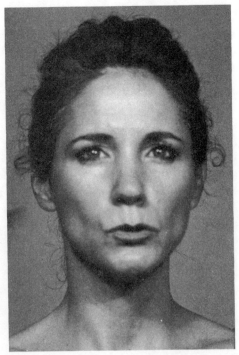

Exercising the oral muscle for fun and beauty.

The oral muscles also give the face an "uplift." They raise the face, raise the upper lip, flare the nostrils, and wrinkle up the nose. They give a happy look to the face.

Esthetic technique: Stroke transversely along the sides of the groove formed by the sides of the nose and the cheek.

Beauty point for acupressure: Center of cheek.

The cranius and triangularis muscles work to push the lips toward the center of the face. They turn the corners of the mouth downward, and in addition draw the corners of the lips to each other. The latter, a triangle-shaped muscle, originates at the chin line, and its fiber extends into the lips. This muscle can cause furrows and pouches in the cheeks and around the mouth, and an expression of sadness.

Exercise: Close your mouth and bite down on your teeth as hard as possible.

Esthetic technique: From the corners of the mouth, stroke down to the neck.

Cheeks

The buccinator muscle controls the cheek. The largest of the oral muscles, it controls blowing, chewing, whistling, and sucking. It also compresses the cheek and retracts the angle of the mouth.

Self technique / exercise: Grit your teeth and apply pressure on the back of the mouth.

Esthetic technique: Locate the area at the corner of the mouth, then stroke it in a straight line out to the ears.

To keep the cheeks from sagging, we must work the muscle that draws the mouth backward and upward. This muscle helps you smile and may cause smile lines. The following techniques will help relieve those lines.

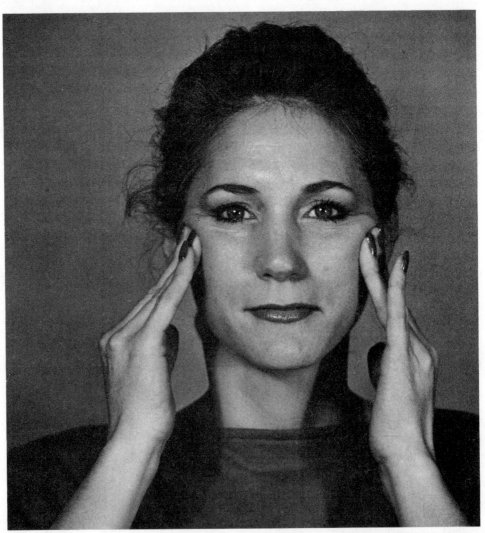

Massaging sagging cheeks. Rotate in small circles while lifting gently toward the eyes.

Exercise: Wink your left eye at least 15 times, then your right, and finally both together. Make sure that you do not move your forehead or mouth as you do so.

Esthetic technique: Find the corner of the mouth and stroke it on an angle up to the ear.

Jaw

The masseter is the great chewing muscle. It is one of the most important facial muscles because it closes the jaw, clenches the teeth when fully contracted, causes the jaw to open and drop, and prevents the cheeks from sagging. Keeping it in good working order can prevent sagging cheeks and TMJ problems. The latter include clenching or grinding of the teeth and a general tightness in the jaw. The temporomandibular joint—where upper and lower jaws meet—is often the site of such problems.

Exercise: Open your mouth wide. (This is sometimes called the lion pose.) Hold the position for about fifteen seconds. Release, and take a deep breath. Repeat at least three times.

Esthetic technique: Apply circular pressure on the side of the face.

Beauty point for acupressure: Along the sides of the face.

Chin

The mentalis is the muscle of the chin that tenses the chin area and also moves the bottom lips. It can cause such facial problems as deep furrows in the chin and sides of the mouth, as well as a double chin.

Self technique: Rub your chin in small circles.

Exercise: Move your mouth from side to side.

Esthetic technique: Apply circular movements on the chin. Then, using the index fingers, gently stroke up toward the mouth.

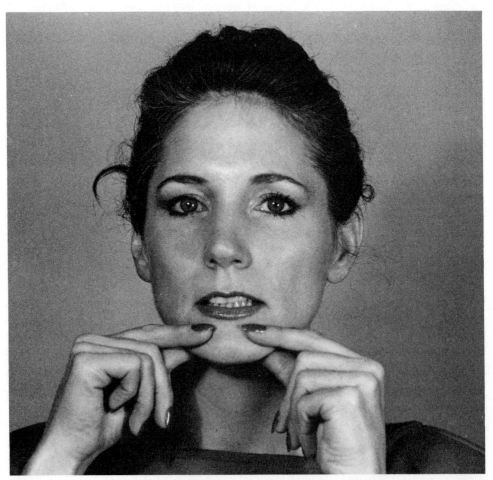

Massaging a double chin. Relax the entire mouth by inhaling, then exhaling the pressure from the mouth and jaw. Let the teeth separate and the mouth relax slightly open. Grasp either side of the chin, gently squeezing following a line along the jawbone. Remember to inhale and exhale during this exercise.

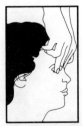

GIVING AN ESTHETIC FACIAL MASSAGE

1. Place both hands on the shoulders and gently hold the back muscles in this area. With a rocking motion, relax the muscles. These muscles are connected to the neck muscles and prepare them to be released.
2. With both hands on the top of the shoulders, gently lean in with the palms, applying slight pressure. Hold for about ten seconds. Repeat three times.
3. Place the palms in front of the shoulders, rock back and forth, then push one side toward the feet. Do the same with the other side.
4. Pick the shoulders up and knead the muscles.
5. Turn the neck to the side. When the large, long muscle in the neck becomes apparent, massage it. Use short, penetrating strokes to slowly rub the neck as you stroke in an upward direction toward the chin. After the short strokes, massage in the same direction, using long, light strokes.
6. Apply circular rhythmic pressure to the base of the chin. Rotate the fingers, covering the entire chin area. Gently massage the chin. With a slight pinching motion, pick the loose skin up and massage toward the lips. Next, use the Dancing Fingers technique to stimulate the circulation in the chin area. Gently tap the fingers over and around the chin. If you notice an indentation in the center of the chin, apply pressure to this area by pressing the line for a period of ten seconds. Repeat three times.
7. As the lips hold a great deal of tension, massaging this area is important. Gently knead the lips, top and bottom.

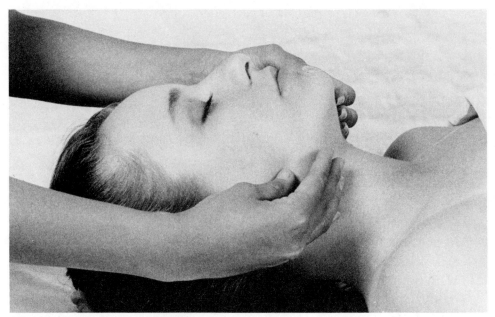

Chin massage during a session.

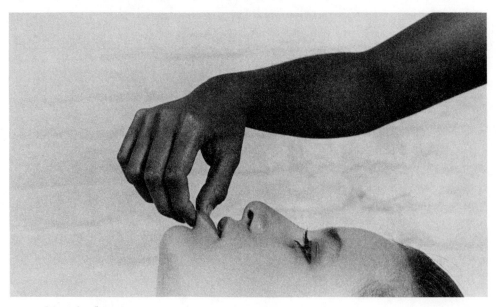

Kneading the lips.

Apply circular strokes to the area. With the index finger, first apply large circular motions. Gradually allow your motions to become smaller and smaller. Begin at the indentation directly under the nostrils, the center point of the lips, and rotate in a clockwise motion around the outer corner of the lips, across the chin and up past the corner of the opposite lip—then back to the center. Rotate in this manner ten times. Next, apply the Dancing Fingers technique around the top and bottom of the lip following the same pattern.

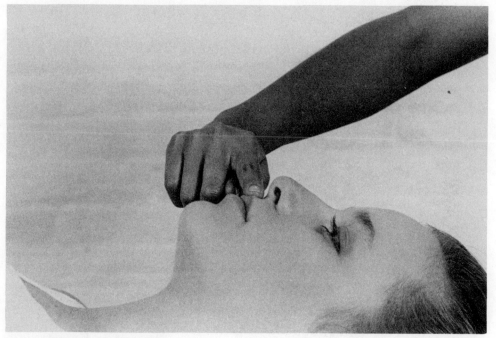

Massaging around the lips.

8. Apply short, quick strokes from the earlobe to the corner of the mouth. Do this on both sides. Next, focus on the area extending from the base of the chin to just behind the earlobes (the space between the corner of the lip and the inside of the lobe). This area we will define as the cheeks. Using long strokes with your index finger, begin with the outer portion of the cheeks closer to the outer ear. Follow the jaw line as you work. Work superior, that is, up toward the ear. Next, move the finger about one-half inch and create an imaginary line as you repeat the direction of your stroke. With your hand on the center of the chin, follow the jaw line with the press-point method.

Specific touch: Press each point slowly and deeply. You will know that you have arrived at the point when you feel some excess energy that may be in the form of a pulsating feeling extending from the chin. When you come to an indentation in the jaw, follow the jaw line. After the very slow and deep strokes, use very long, deep pressure. Take your time and move slowly. Next, use very long and light strokes.

9. Massage behind the ear, using short strokes up toward the ear. When you reach the ear, go to the outside of it and, again using short strokes, work back to the ear. Repeat this until you reach the area about one inch from the eye.

10. Now, we are at the eye. Eye massage has many benefits, especially for tired eyes that may feel heavy and for increasing the circulation around the auricular area. The eye, when it is under strain, will become puffy, or the skin may become extremely loose and lose its firmness and tone. Sagging eyebrows or eyelids as well as unwanted lines under and on the side of the eye may also occur.

With the hands about three inches to either side of the eye, rotate the finger in a circular motion following the natural direction of the eyebrow hair. First, rotate in large circles. Follow the pattern approximately three inches above the eye, working down toward the eyelash. When you reach the bottom of the eyelash, stop and repeat this motion two more times. Rotate ten times in each direction. Remember, the eye contains very soft, sensitive tissues that can be damaged if the pressure applied is too hard or too prolonged. Also

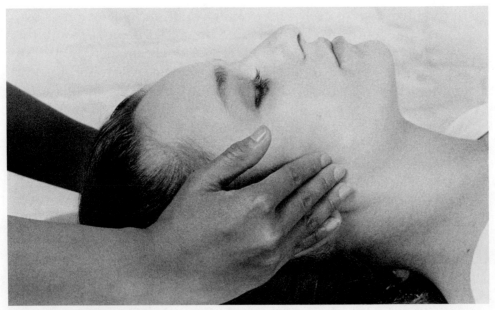

The cheeks and the jaw.

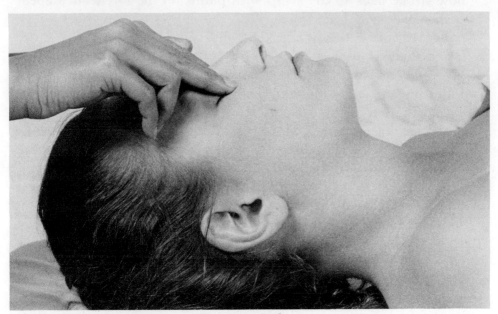

Massaging the eyes. Be sure to be very gentle.

be careful of the eye itself. Make your circular movements very slow, so that you control your fingers and do not let them slip onto the eye. After your circles have gotten progressively smaller and you've reached the eyebrow, lightly "dance" your fingers around the eye and under-eye, creating stimulation and circulation in this area. Next, place your fingers at the bottom corner of each nostril and with very long but slow strokes, massage the area from the nostril up over the eyebrows, following the face's natural path.

The corner of the nostrils contain a very precious body oil. You may put this oil back into the skin by rubbing it on the forehead. As you stroke, move from the corner of the nostril up over the eyebrows three times and then take slow, short strokes moving only about one inch each time. Once you have taken one inch, move the fingers up another inch. Continue until you have reached the top of the eyebrows.

11. With the palms flat on the forehead, stroke back, allowing the fingers to trail toward the back of the neck. From the top of the eyebrow, now stroke back to the scalp with palms on the forehead. Repeat each movement three times. With the fingers on the cheeks, lean back with the entire hand. Next, slide the hands down the entire face and the sides.

12. When you arrive at the area around the corner of the eye, using the index finger, slowly move in a straight line from the corner of the eye to the top of the earlobe. Next, use long deep strokes on this area, stroking ten times. Move behind the ear and repeat, following the contour of the muscle to the point where it ends, stroke the back of the scalp toward the base of the neck.

Massage the ears, grasping them gently between the index finger and the thumb, at the top of the lobe. Follow the circle of the ear until you have reached the lobe. Use slight and gentle circular, rhythmic pressure—still with the lobe between the index finger and the thumb—to massage the lobe.

13. It is now time to apply the special beauty points. These are six specially located areas of the face that may have as their focus some

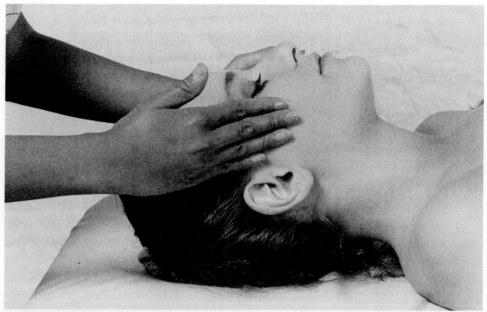

Following the facial contour.

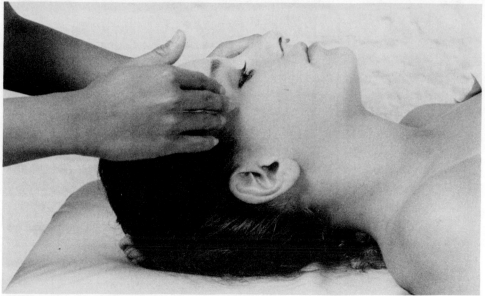

The forehead and scalp.

activity or action that will prompt facial stimulation. By applying pressure to these points, you will bring good coloration and skin tone to this area. Some of the points are coordinated with muscles, while others have their own location and pathways. The special beauty points should not be approached with forcefulness. Instead, lean gently into the points, applying pressure for about fifteen seconds, releasing, and then repeating two more times.

Point #1—Locate the point that lies directly in the center, or cleft, of the chin. You will know the point by an indentation or slight groove that invites your finger to touch there. Apply pressure for about fifteen seconds and repeat three times.

Point #2—Apply slight pressure to the corner of each lip, holding approximately fifteen seconds, then releasing. Repeat this three times. When you arrive at the corner of the lip, the beauty point is just on the inside.

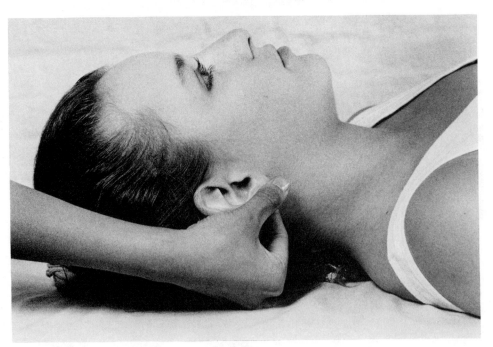

Gentle, circular pressure to the earlobes.

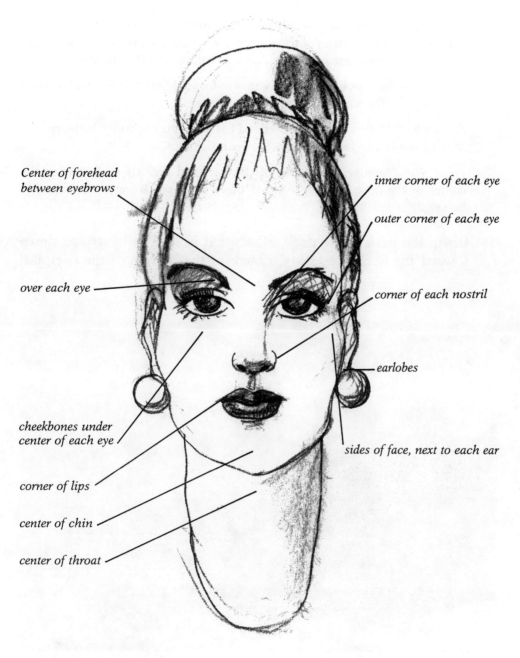

Center of forehead
between eyebrows

inner corner of each eye

outer corner of each eye

over each eye

corner of each nostril

earlobes

cheekbones under
center of each eye

sides of face, next to each ear

corner of lips

center of chin

center of throat

The face's beauty points.

Point #3—Looking straight ahead, line your finger up with the center of the eye just at the corner of the nostril. Here you will find a special beauty point that brings tone and stimulates circulation in the cheeks.

Point #4—The special beauty points are located between the eyebrows in the center of the forehead and over each eye.

Point #5—The center of the forehead between the eyebrows helps reduce scowl lines in the forehead and between the eyes.

Point #6—Massage the center of the forehead directly in line with the center of the nose, moving toward the scalp (approximately two inches below it).

14. Grasp the back of the neck. Massage it in long, firm strokes down toward the back. Repeat. Go back to the bottom of the occipital

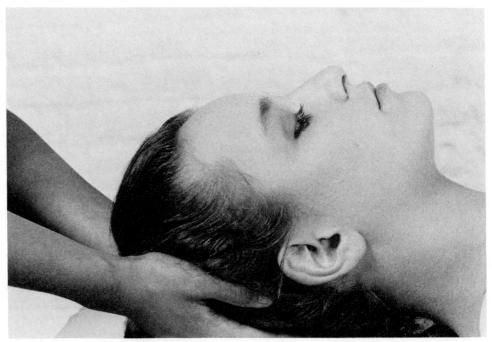

Stroking the back of the neck.

bone (just above the end of the hairline) and apply a circular, rhythmic pressure. Apply touch along the line of the occipital bone. Now, continue the strokes from the occipital area to the back. Stroke each part ten times.

15. Rub the hands together until you feel a sort of heat, then gently lay the palm of the hand over the eye, cupping the entire face. As you do so, make light, feathery strokes from the chin up toward the head. Repeat this for about two minutes.

16. Use the Dancing Fingers technique over the entire face. Stay in each spot at least ten seconds, tapping the fingers very slowly and lightly, thereby increasing the circulation to each area. Rub the hands together again and when you feel heat between them, place them over the entire face.

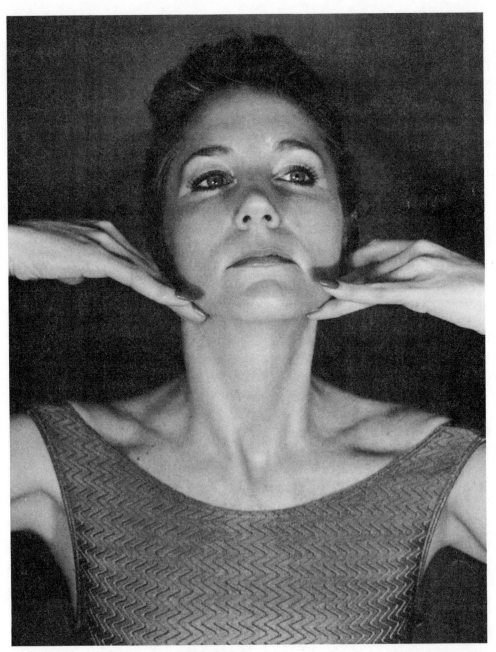

A well-toned neck is a beautiful thing.

6

Hold Your Head High: Throat and Neck

The muscles of the neck give support and form to the throat, which houses the voice. They function as a connecting bridge between the head, chest, and shoulders. Discomfort in the voice can be related to muscles in the neck. The internal muscles control the opening and closing of vocal folds, as well as the voice's pitch. Pitch quality can be manipulated as well as voice tone. The amount of air that passes through the neck is generated internally.

Below is a list of neck-related difficulties that can be helped by massage:

- flabby neck
- irritated throat
- poor voice quality
- inability to speak up and express oneself
- neck cramp
- laryngitis
- torticollis
- whiplash

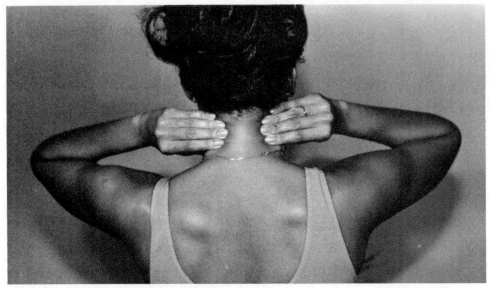

Massaging under the occipital bone relieves tension, tones muscles, and increases circulation in the back of the neck

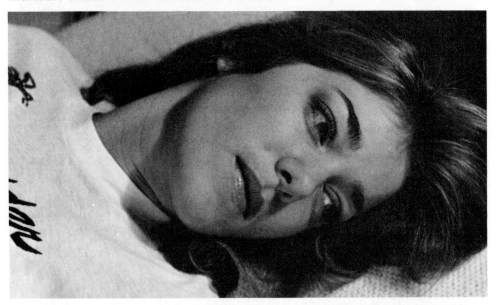

Stretching the neck. Lying on your back, move your head from side to side as far as is comfortable.

Self techniques:

1. On your stomach: Grasp the spot under the occiput and squeeze in from both sides.
2. Sitting in a chair: Place both hands, folded, behind your head. Lean into your hands, resisting with your head.
3. Bend over and simply drop your neck, letting the tension fall from your shoulders. Place your hands on the seventh cervical vertebra (the large, protruding knob at the base of the neck) and use the Dancing Fingers technique.
4. Stretching the neck: Visualize that a balloon, tied to a string and attached to your head, is pulling your head and neck straight up. Feel your entire body stand erect.

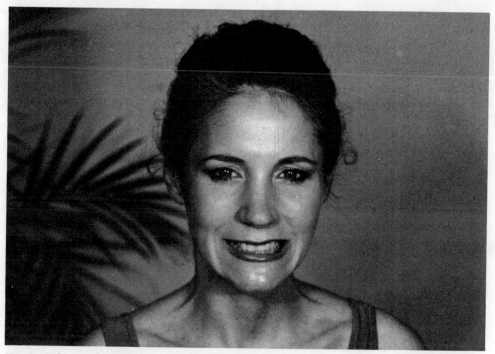

Toning the neck muscles. Create a large grin involving the use of the neck muscles and the lower facial muscles. Hold the tension for a few seconds, then exhale as you release.

Exercises:
1. Hold the neck upright; rotate slowly in both directions.
2. Stick the tongue out as far as possible. Curl the tongue at the end so it reaches toward the nose.
3. Place the hands on the sides of the head with the thumb and index finger on either side of the ear. Raise the head.
4. Grasp the spot under the occiput, lean back gently, and apply circular pressure.
5. In the tub, relax and visualize the neck stretching.

Esthetic technique:
With a gliding motion grasp the neck with clasped hands, one on each side. Stroke from the bottom of the chin to the bottom of the neck.

These are some techniques and exercises you can use to aid in toning, relaxing, and relieving the throat area. Remember that a positive attitude will help produce a beautiful neck!

7

Shoulders and Arms

The shoulders are a unique part of the body. They offer support for the neck and head, and consist of a shallow ball-and-socket joint that is highly prone to injury. A shoulder is held intact by ligaments, joint capsules, tendons, nerves, lymph, muscles, and bones. Bursitis and stiffness are common in this area.

The following constitute the muscles of the shoulder:

- Deltoid: This muscle forms the round area of the shoulder and the upper arm.
- Trapezius: This muscle raises the shoulders. It is superficial and lies immediately under the connective tissue. It elevates the shoulders. Both trapezius muscles help stabilize the shoulders when carrying something heavy. They also play a part in shrugging the shoulders.
- Serratus anterior: This muscle raises the shoulder.

The shoulder is subject to the following conditions: stiffness; tightness; drooping and sagging; spasm (irregular pulsation in the muscle, alternating between contraction and expansion).

Self techniques: Squeeze the shoulders. (Begin at joint and work to neck.)
Knead the shoulders.

Exercises: Rotate shoulders.
Lift barbells straight up.
Turn neck to the right, while turning the shoulders to the left.

Esthetic technique: Place hand in scapula, with arms folded across the back. Gently push.
Knead the shoulder.
Rotate the shoulder.

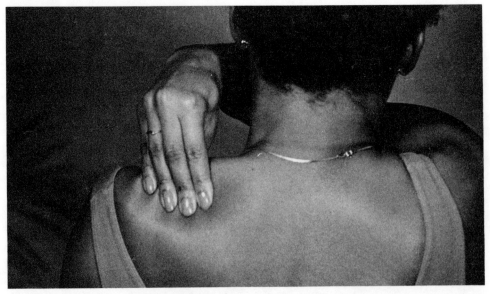

Kneading the shoulder and arm joint.

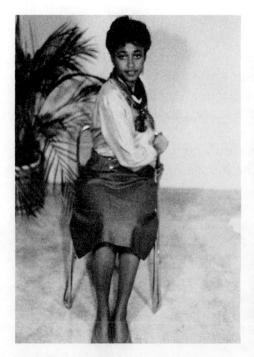 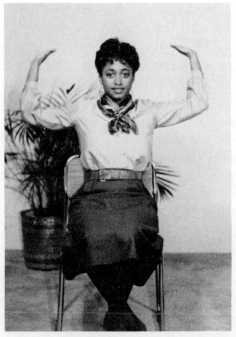

Slowly turning the neck and shoulders in opposite directions.

Stretching the shoulders. Reach back with both arms over the head, giving the shoulder blades a good stretch. Feel the benefits as you release the tension and tightness.

Push the shoulders toward feet.
Knead the neck.
Knead the arm.

Between the shoulder and the hand there is . . . the arm. The upper arm extends from the shoulder girdle to the elbow. Eleven muscles operate it to produce a wide variety of movements:

Flexion is the bending of a joint between the bones of a limb, by which the angle between the bones is diminished (i.e., raising the arm forward).

Extension is the unbending of a joint between the bones of a limb, by which the angle of the bones is increased (i.e., lowering the arm).

Abduction is the moving of a limb away from the body.

Adduction is the moving of a limb toward the body.

Circumduction is the rotation or circular motion of a limb.

Many of the muscles in the forearm are responsible for manipulating the hand.

Some of the common discomforts in the arm include: tennis elbow; arthritis; bursitis (inflammation of the bursae in the shoulder); limited range of motion.

If the arms are well exercised and stimulated, the muscles will not deteriorate to the point of weakness and aching.

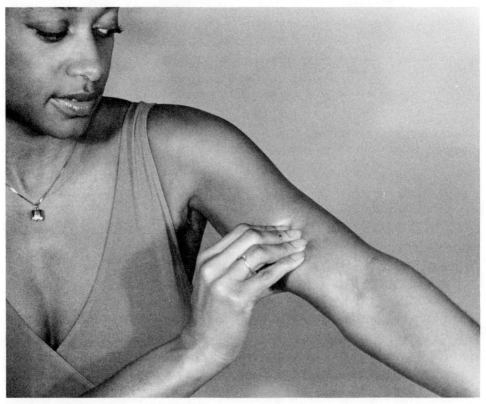

Kneading biceps for tone in arms.

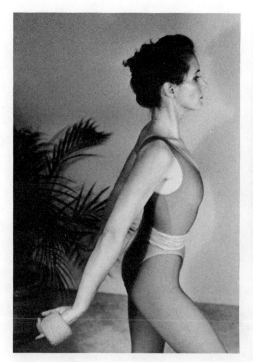

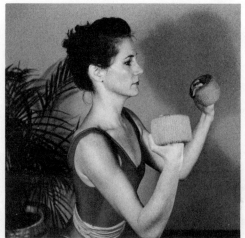

Curling and stretching with moderate weights improves muscle tone and posture.

Self technique: Lock your fingers and stretch them overhead.

Exercises:
Strengthening, weights, curls.
Range of motion.
Wrist rotation.

Esthetic techniques:
Kneading.
Stretching, traction.
Overhead, folding of arms.

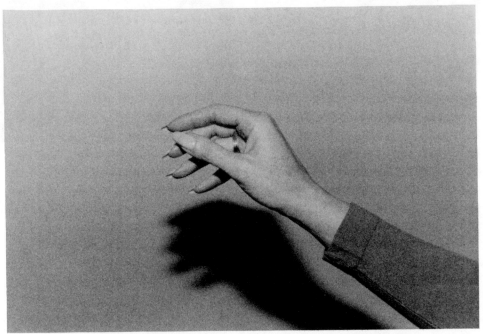

Proper exercise and massage can give you relaxed, graceful hands.

8

With a Loving Touch: Hands

The hand is one of the most remarkable parts of the human body. It serves as a fine sense organ (i.e., serving to discern temperatures and sharpness) and as a tool capable of delicate manipulations. Its many nerve endings enable us to determine the texture and shape of objects we have not seen.

The hand's mobility results from the diversity of joints in the upper arm. Muscles in the wrist and arm also help give the hand further variety of movement.

Some problems of the hand are: arthritis; writer's cramp; dull sense of touch; numbness in fingers; coldness due to poor circulation; nails that crack or break; inability to bend fingers.

In almost every expression the body makes, the hands are involved at some level. Hands bear the tension from anger or fear, which causes them to be tightly clenched. In surprise or elation, by contrast, they are relaxed and open, with the arms also usually thrown open and back.

Self techniques:

1. Grasp the tip of your finger. Keeping the hand stationary, rotate the finger, first clockwise, then counterclockwise. Do the same for each finger, making sure you touch each one firmly. Sometimes just feeling the presence of our beautiful hands provides a special self-awareness.

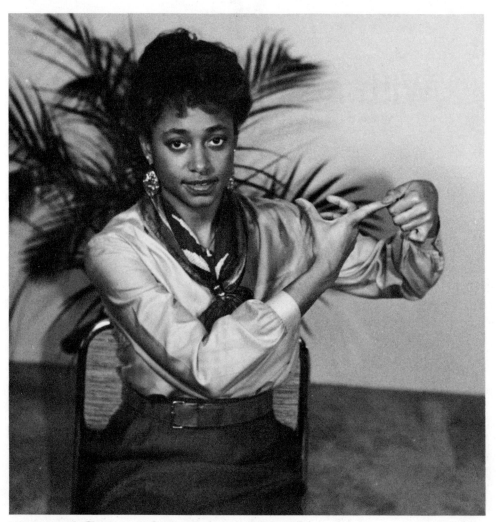

Rotate each finger to relieve stress in your hands.

2. Rotate your hand by grasping the fingers of the opposite hand. Twist it slightly, becoming aware of any tightness or tension as you rotate.

3. There is a special reflex point for headache and neck tension in the hand. To locate the point, place the first groove of your thumb (the first line across the thumb, on the palm side) at the top of the area between the index finger and thumb (this will be the area where lighter and darker skin meet). Let the thumb fall naturally and apply pressure in the area most sensitive to the touch (see pressure-point diagram for the hand).

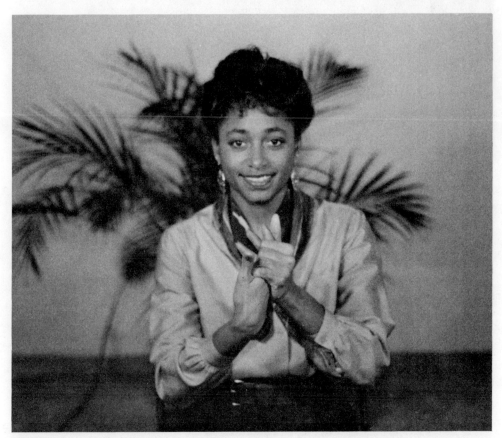

Rotate the wrist and hand to find specific areas of high tension.

Exercises:
Use weights and barbells to strengthen the hands. Also, squeeze a
rubber ball to build strength and release tension.

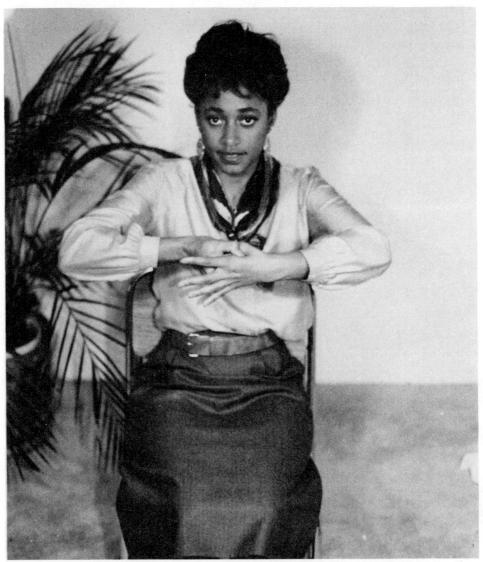

Finding and massaging the special headache relief point in the hand.

(Back of hands)

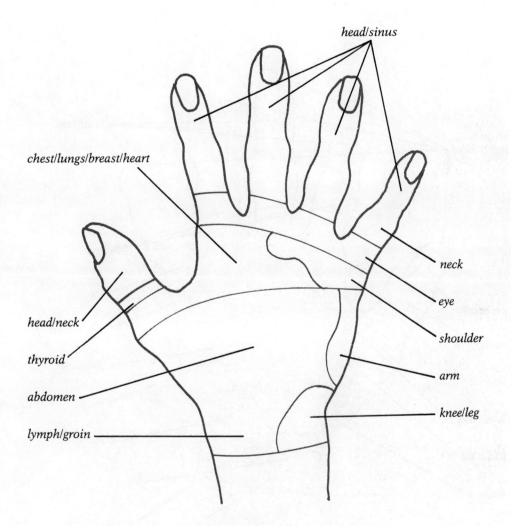

head/sinus

chest/lungs/breast/heart

neck

eye

shoulder

head/neck

thyroid

arm

abdomen

knee/leg

lymph/groin

Organ-related pressure points in the left and right hands.

(Front left hand)

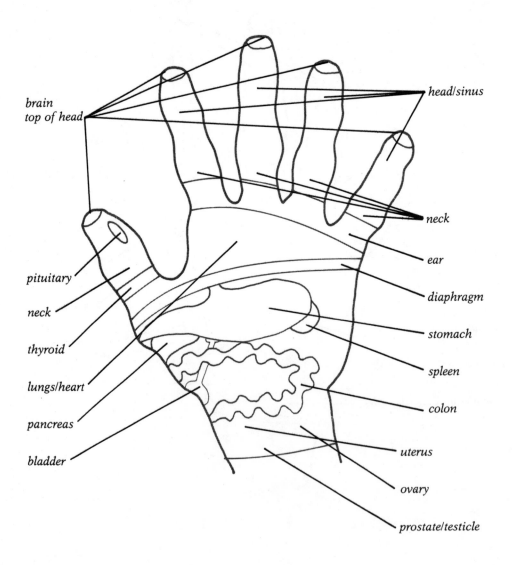

Organ-related pressure points in the left hand.

(Front right hand)

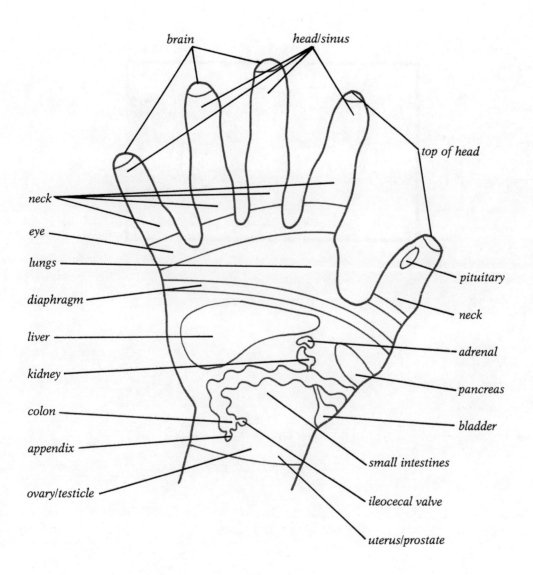

Organ-related pressure points in the right hand.

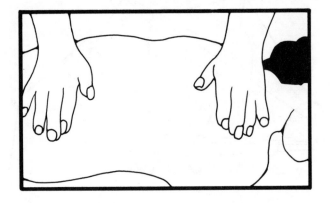

9

Chest Out, Stomach In: Posture and Chest

Posture: the way you stand, the way you sit, the way you walk, the positions your body moves to. Each of these activities helps shape your body's contour. Proper alignment can help prevent aches and pains. One thing is for sure: The better your posture, the better you will feel about yourself.

The way in which you hold your body affects your mental attitudes. What do the following say about the way you feel?

- Head hung high
- Head hung low
- Shoulders dropped
- Chest stuck out like a peacock
- Arms and legs constantly tightly crossed
- Fists constantly clenched

Slumping may seem to take the pressure off a weak muscle, but it actually stresses it and affects some other muscle that is offering support for it. Good posture takes pressure off the spine and distributes it evenly throughout the body.

Moving posture is involved when we perform some given action.

For example, when we walk many different muscles are called into action. The feet go up, down, and forward. The waist moves from side to side. The arms swing back and forth. The hands open and close. The neck goes up and down, as the shoulders cause the chest to expand, which in turn moves the neck. We inhale and exhale, which also creates movement.

The object of moving posture is to insure a smooth, stress-free movement to each stride. If a bad habit is allowed to set in, it will soon become hard to correct. When it is repeated over and over, a slump, pain, wrinkle, or other unwanted appearance may occur. In the proper beauty or fitness routine, good posture should be practiced even away from the spa or health club.

Here are some helpful things to consider when examining your overall posture as you stand facing a mirror:

- Is one shoulder higher than the other?
- Is one leg turned in more than the other?
- Is your head hanging down or is your body supporting it, upright?
- Is the chest area open, or are the shoulders crowding it by being turned in?
- Is your back hunched or slumped over?
- Are your fists clenched?
- Is there tension in your face?
- Are your toes turned upward?

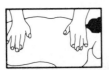

CHESTS AND BREASTS ARE IN!

The way you carry your chest says a lot about you. If your chest is sunken (not due to structural imbalance) and your shoulders are dropped, it is possible you don't give the impression that you feel good about yourself. Make sagging breasts and flat chests a thing of the past: Stand tall!

Massage can be beneficial to help alleviate bronchitis and chest muscle spasms, to strengthen a sunken chest, and restore suppleness to breasts.

Often curvatures of the spine will cause distortions in the chest; many of these can be compensated for by good posture and exercise.

Self technique:

To stimulate circulation and energy flow in the chest, apply circular pressure to a point just below the breast. The technique is doubly effective when the corresponding point just above the breast is massaged as well. Locate the points just above and below the nipple. Hold for a few seconds and release, then repeat.

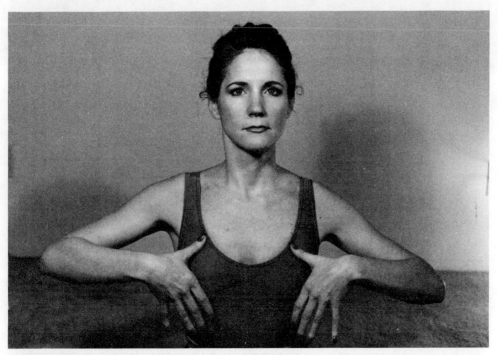

Applying pressure to special points in the chest.

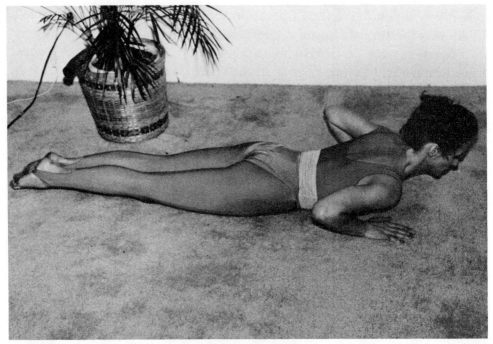

Push-ups will strengthen and tone the entire body.

Exercises:
Push-ups will tone and relax muscles in the chest and breast, as
   well as the upper arms and abdomen. Exhale as you bend your
   arms, and inhale as you push yourself back up.

Esthetic technique:
To stimulate the respiratory system, open the chest, and counteract
   slumping shoulders, grasp the hands and place them behind the
   head. Place your hands on the receiver's folded arms and lean
   back, pulling gently on the arms in either direction. Feels great!

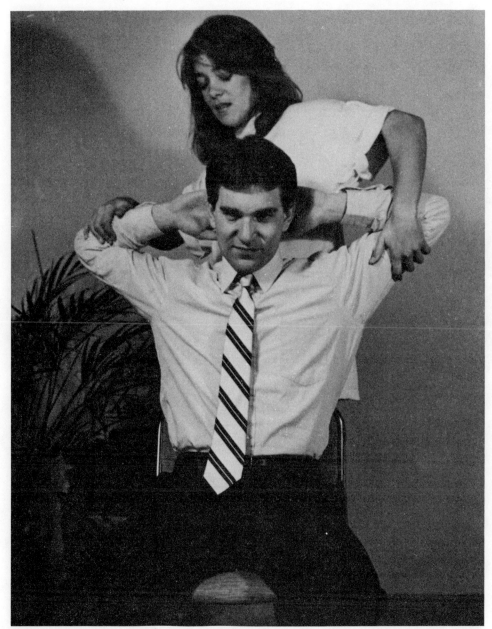

Esthetic massage to open and stimulate the entire chest and respiratory system.

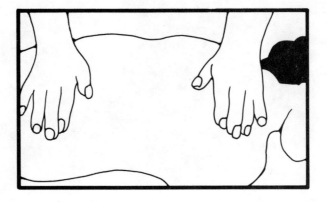

10

Backs Are Beautiful Too!

Entire books have been written about the back and about ways of relieving the nagging pain that so many people experience. Muscles in the back tighten before any other muscles. In addition, the back is a sort of receptacle, in that it is sent tension from other parts of the body. So don't forget about the back: When it receives massage, it feels gooood!

The main muscles in the back are:

- Deltoid—lifts the arm
- Infrasinatus—rotates the humerus laterally
- Teres major—rotates the arm laterally
- Teres minor—adducts the arm, extends and rotates the arm to the center of the body
- Quadratus lumborum—Flexes the lumbar vertebrae laterally
- Spinal cervicis—extends the vertebral column

- Latissimus dorsi ("lats")—adducts and extends the arm to the center of the body
- Trapezius—rotates the scapula to raise the shoulder, adducts the arm, and draws scapula backward
- Gluteus maximus—extends, abducts, and rotates the thigh laterally
- Adductor magnus—adducts the thigh; the superficial part extends the thigh
- Semitendinous—flexes the leg and extends the thigh

More people experience back discomfort than any other single ailment. There are several causes:

- Structural imbalance (one leg longer, etc.)
- Mental stress and emotional worries
- Lifting heavy loads
- Structural problems (lordosis, etc.)
- Lack of muscle tone
- Weak stomach muscles
- Weak back muscles
- Bad posture
- Wearing high heels too often
- Sitting too long

Back discomfort is usually felt in the lower segment. This is not to say that other areas do not experience it, but the lower back is especially vulnerable. When massage is applied to this area, it relaxes the entire body. While relaxing it, it also stimulates the brain's so-called pleasure center, which is responsible for sending and receiving signals related to pleasure. An initial feeling of total calmness is felt, followed by a new sense of vitality.

The back has its own network of message centers located in the spine. The spinal cord has nerve connections to just about every part of the body. Thus, every part of the body can receive a sensation from the back area. Standing upright, with an air of "feeling good" about oneself, adds dramatically to one's personal beauty.

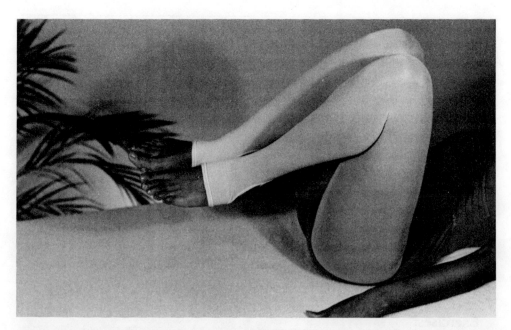

Tried-and-true relief for lower-back tension.

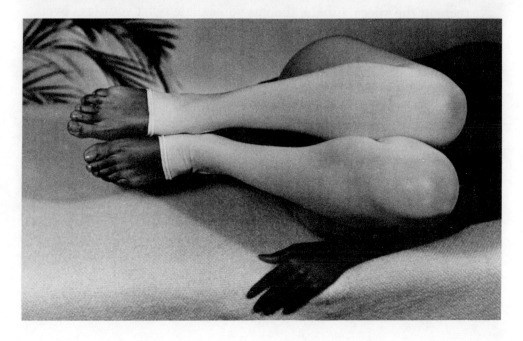

> Lordosis—also called swayback—is caused by an anterior cavity in the curvature of the spine. The compensatory curve will be found in the cervical spine area.
>
> Flat back is a lumbar curve with less sway than lordosis.
>
> Kyphosis is the round back condition seen in hunchbacks.
>
> Scoliosis is a lateral curvature of the spine.

Self technique: Lie flat on your stomach. Gradually lift your legs up from the floor, followed gradually by your chest. Soon you will feel the pressure on your lower, middle, or upper back. When the pressure reaches the desired spot, hold the position for a count of 10. Gradually release.

Exercises:

1. Lower back—Lie flat on the floor. Slowly lift your legs, bending them at the knees. Inhale, then as you exhale twist your legs over to the right. You will feel a slight tension in the lower back. Move your legs as close to the floor as possible, then raise them to the starting point, where you began. Repeat several times. Alleviates a tight and tense lower back.

2. Upper back—Sitting in a chair, grasp the back of one side of the chair with both hands. Twisting only your back, inhale and turn to the side of the chair you are holding, as far as possible. As you exhale, turn your upper body even farther.

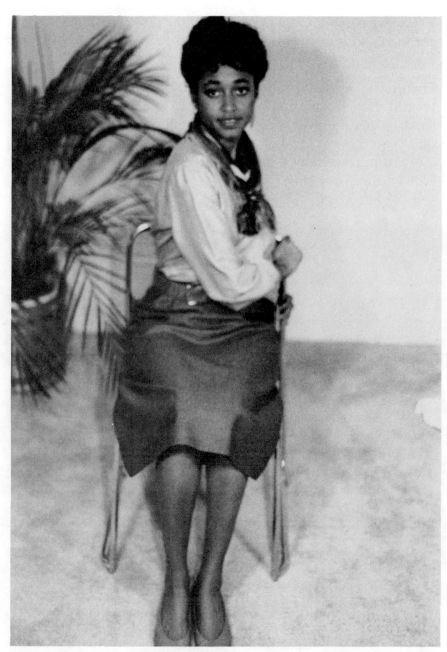

Twist slowly, but as far as possible, to ease tension in the upper back.

3. Entire back—In a sitting position on the floor, cross one leg over the other. Place your hands solidly on the floor, then turn your body to the opposite direction.

4. Energizing spine and entire back—Sitting in a chair, take a deep breath and slowly allow your body to fall forward, until your hands touch the floor. Stay in this position for a few moments. Close your eyes and release the tension by visualizing it flowing away from your body. Inhale deeply and take a long exhalation. Slowly raise your body.

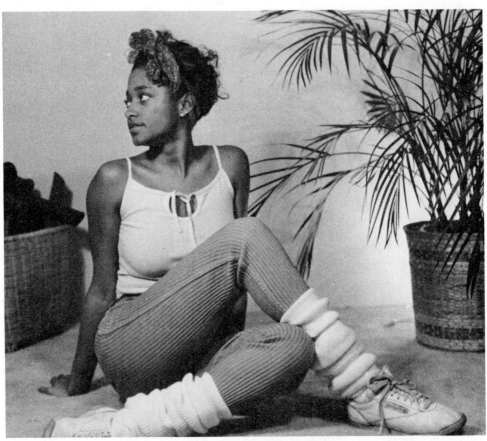

More twisting and turning to relax your back and improve your posture.

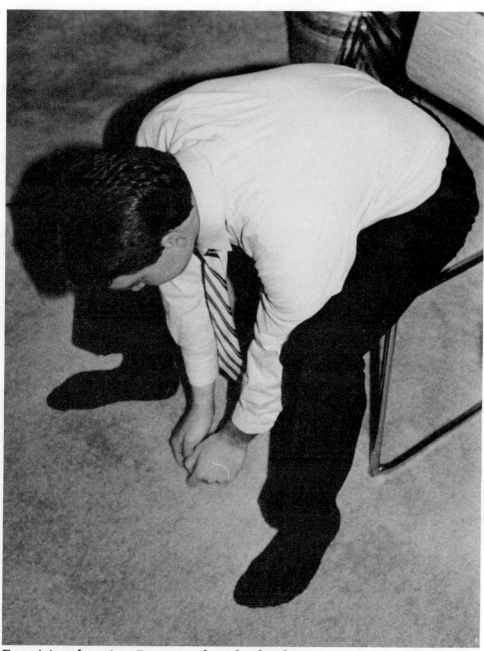

Energizing the spine. Be sure to breathe deeply.

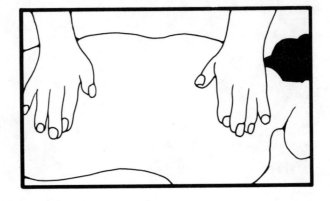

11

Abdomen and Pelvis

The abdomen and pelvis constitute the lower portion of the trunk. They equal the feet in importance in maintaining proper balance and posture.

Subcutaneous connective tissue in most parts of the body consists of a single layer whose thickness depends on its fat content. In the abdomen there are two, three, or four layers of fat. The surface layer consists of one of the body's major fat deposits. It may be more than 1 inch thick. The lower layer supports a fatty layer and helps skin move. No wonder it's so easy to get a ring around the tummy!

Beauty problems in the abdomen and pelvis can include: stretch marks; a beer belly; cellulite; unshapely hips and thighs. Other problems may take the form of upset stomach and bloatedness, as well as menstrual cramps and tense inner organs.

The following are common disorders in this area that are helped by massage:

- Constipation—use abdominal massage and hot packs on the lower back.

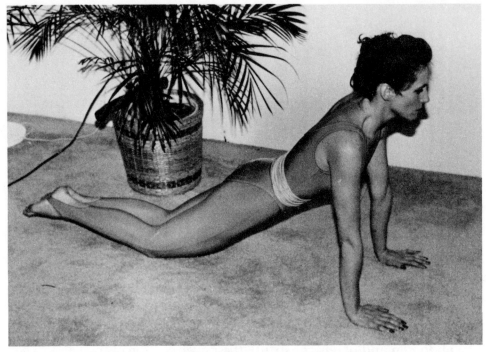

Leg and chest lifts. They're strenuous but very gratifying!

- Gastritis (inflammation of the stomach wall)—deep breathing and gentle stomach massage may help relieve discomfort.
- Hemorrhoids (varicosed or dilated blood vessels around the anal area)—apply deep massage to the lower back.

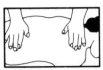

ABDOMINAL EXERCISES

Abdominal breathing is one of the best ways to relieve tension, tightness, or discomfort in the abdominal area. Stomach cramps, indigestion, or

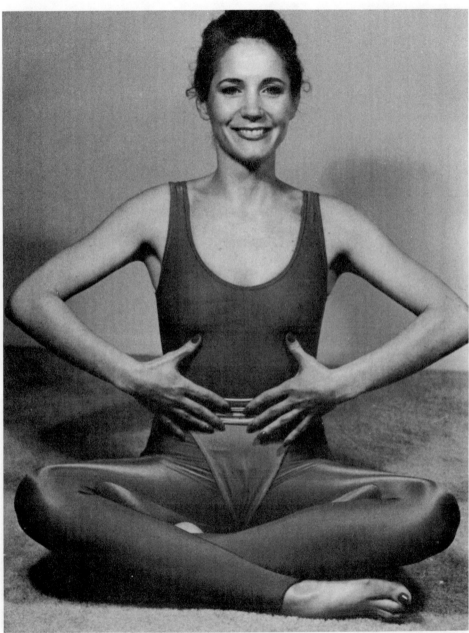

Sit with your back very straight and breathe deeply, into and out of the abdomen.

tight muscles are also helped by this technique. Simply sit with your back and spine as straight as possible. Make sure there are no disturbances as you exercise. Focus on the area around your navel by first placing your hands over this area to direct the energy. Now begin inhaling deeply. Pretend you are breathing into your hands, trying to make the stomach area expand like a balloon. Then hold your breath for a few seconds. When you release the breath, exhale twice as slow as you inhaled. Repeat this at least three times, each time breathing deeper, and exhaling at a slower pace.

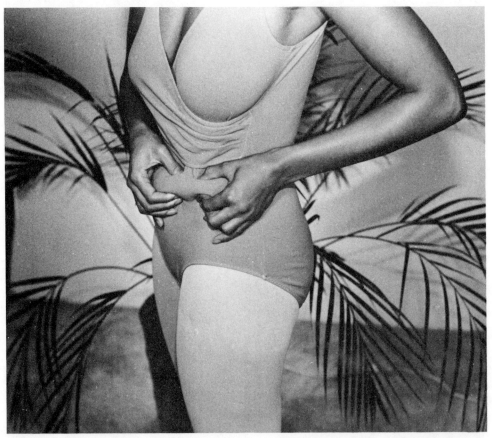

Kneading the tummy. Repeat this exercise a few times each day for a trimmer, shapelier waistline.

Self techniques:

Grasp an area on the side of the waist between your four fingers and the thumb. Lightly knead this area for a few seconds. This technique releases tension and tightness and improves circulation to this area. Repeat in a circular motion, around the entire stomach area. Then pull the skin out, as you release vital energies from the skin surface.

Lie on your back. Breathe into your abdomen. Gently rub the entire area in a circular motion. Begin at the navel and work in a clockwise direction. When you have again reached the navel area, begin again. This time, however, apply a light pressure, as you gently press in on the stomach. Again, press lightly, all over, in a clockwise motion.

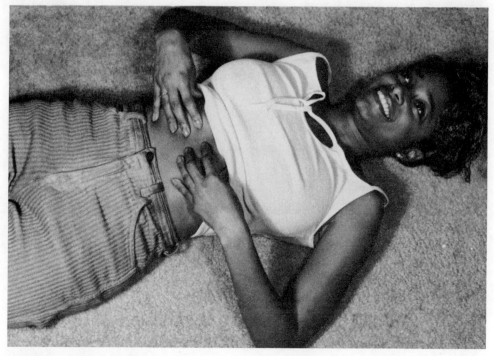

Waking up the tummy.

TOWEL MASSAGE

Stretching and massaging with a towel is like dancing: Just follow the lead of your body and it will show you the next step.

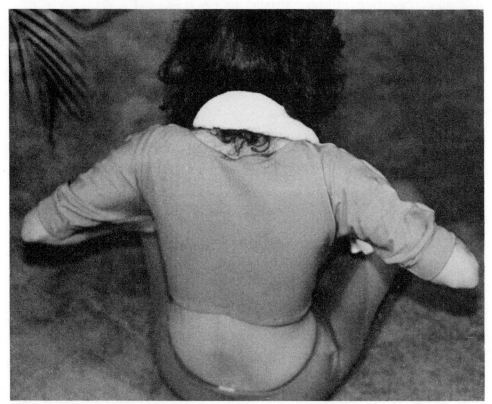

Place the towel behind the neck. Roll it back and forth to get the same effect as in rubbing or kneading the muscle.

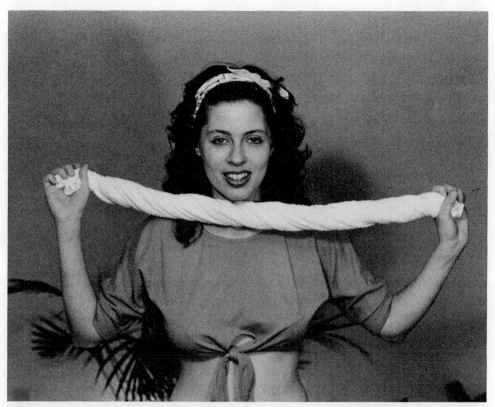

Place it under the chin and push up. Push the entire head and face up. Hold for a few seconds, then release.

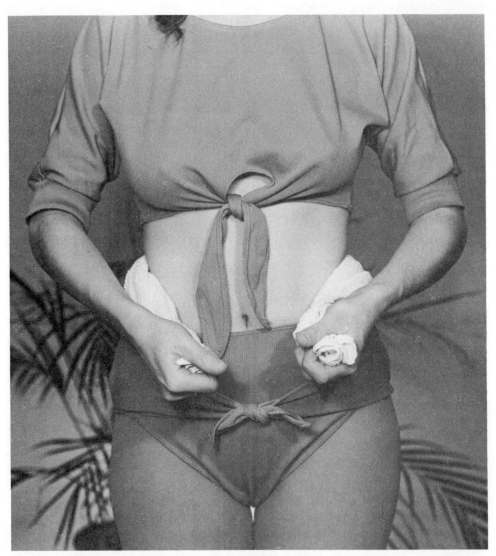

Fighting cellulite and trimming the waistline. Wrap the towel around the back and pull it tight. This works the lower back.

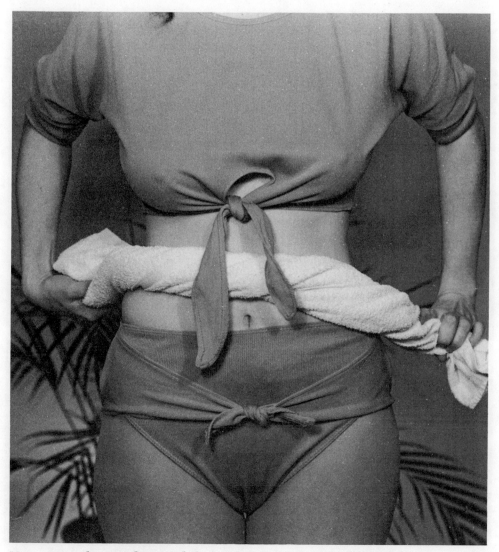

Now, wrap the towel around the entire stomach and pull it back and forth.

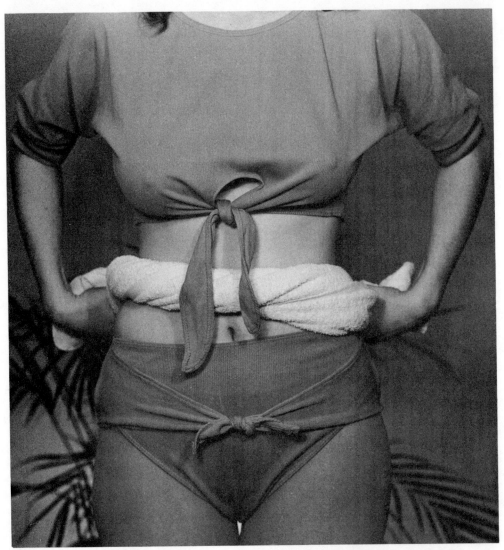

Next, move the towel to the front of the stomach and pull it toward the back.

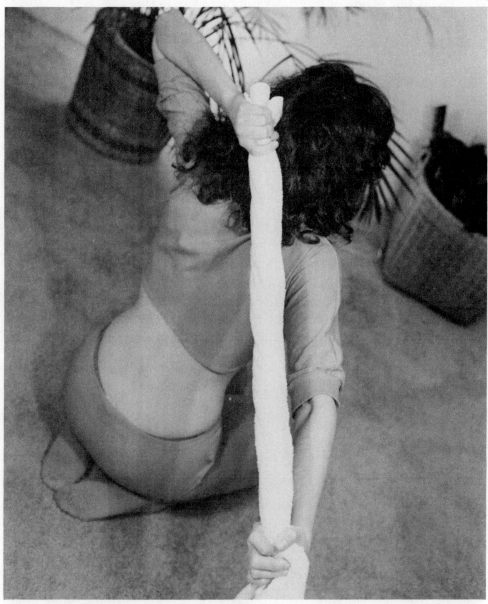

Toning back and shoulder muscles. Hold the towel around the neck and pull down toward the feet. Hold for a few seconds and release.

The pelvis is one of the most important structures in the body and perhaps the most neglected. It acts as the balance between the top and bottom and between the left and right sides. Otherwise known as the hip bone, it is formed from two bones separated by the tailbone and the sacrum. It is the lowermost part of the spine. As the lowest portion of the trunk, it marks the beginning of the lower body. Without the pelvis, the sexual organs, the bladder, colon, and buttocks would not have support. They are all housed in this area. Because of childbirth, the female pelvis is slightly different in structure from the male pelvis. It may be larger in body proportion and less curved. It is also a very sensitive location. When most people—male or female—are touched in this area, there is an emotional reaction of some kind.

In determining posture, the pelvic girdle is important. It acts as a support and balancer very much the way the collar bone does. It balances the abdomen that balances the shoulders that balance the neck and head.

Since sexual organs carry an energy of their own, when pelvic structure is out of line, their function will be hindered. A stomach that hangs excessively, an abnormally arched back, weak lower back muscles, and drooped shoulders will all take away from your vital energy. Correction of these conditions begins with alignment of the pelvic area.

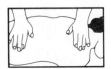

PELVIC EXERCISES

Pelvic dip: Lie flat on your stomach. With your knees on the floor, raise your body at the waist. Lower your waist to the floor, and raise it up again. You will be taking deep dips with your stomach, in a sort of pelvic push-up activity.

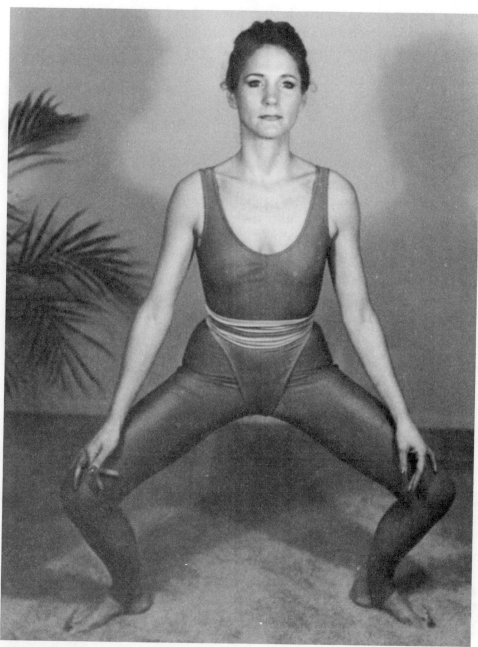

Riding the Horse.

Pelvic stretch: Lie on your side. Place your hand firmly on the floor. Lift one leg, and stretch it as far as you can. Hold this position for a few seconds. Repeat three times and then repeat with the other leg.

Riding the Horse: Stand erect. Inhale, and slowly bend the knees as if you were riding a horse. Hold this position for a moment, then exhale. Inhale and dip even farther, each time opening the pelvis a bit more. When you have stretched as far as you can, return and begin again. This unblocks sexual energies and loosens tight pelvic muscles.

Self technique: Locate the pelvic points to either side of the hip bone. Apply gently circular massage to the point for a period of ten to fifteen seconds. Repeat three times.

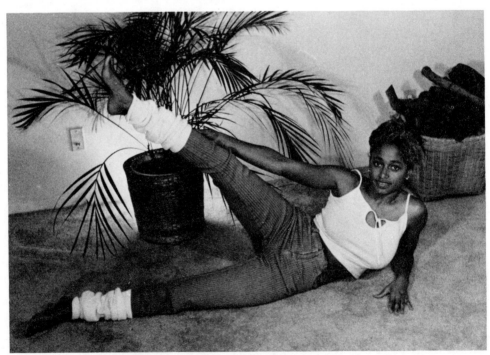

Leg lifts to stimulate and strengthen the pelvis.

12

Legs

The area between the pelvis and the knees is properly known as the thigh, while the area between the feet and the knees is properly known as the leg. However, the total area, including the lower leg, knees, thigh, and buttocks, is usually called the leg. Massage can benefit the leg and give it shape, form, and smoothness.

The buttocks, which are formed by a rounded mass of gluteal muscle, are a resting place and sort of a landing platform. They usually hold discomfort from other parts of the body and thus constitute a very sensitive area. Discomfort may arise in the thighs from contracted muscles on the opposite side of the thighs. Remember that muscles work like a pulley system. When one muscle becomes too tight, the opposite muscle will stretch to compensate. Eventually the stretched muscle will lose its tone and elasticity. This will result in flabby skin, or even stretch marks in the thigh area.

Common leg problems include: sports injuries; stiff knee; housewife's knee; rough skin; weakness; varicose veins; cellulite.

Massage will give legs a more shapely appearance and help with the above conditions. The following are my special recommendations for beautiful legs.

Self techniques:

Locate the pressure point on the side of your knee (where the indentation is felt). Apply gentle, then deep pressure to this point. This stimulates circulation in the legs.

   Locate the pressure point on the back of your leg by raising your foot to place the pressure on your toes, and finding the muscle which protrudes. The point is just below this muscle. Apply gentle, then deep pressure to this point. This will relieve tight and tired leg muscles.

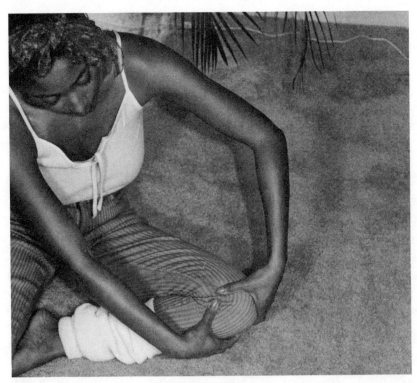

Massaging the pressure point inside the knee.

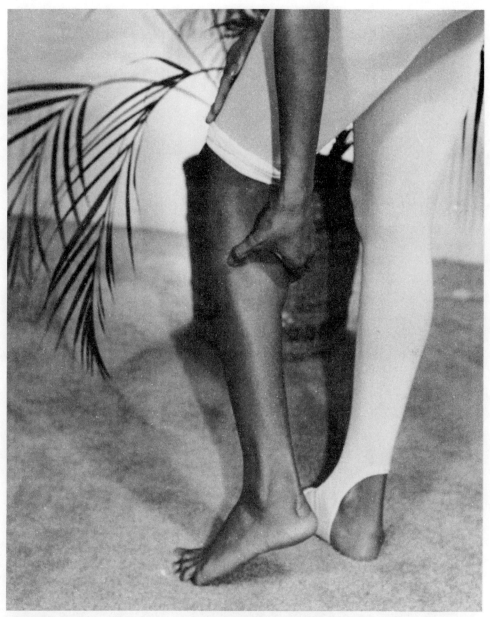

Kneading the calf muscle—a runner's delight! Calf muscles are involved in every step we take, and, especially for those who take many steps—dancers, runners, salespeople—this technique brings great joy.

Exercise:

Sit with one leg crossed and the other stretched out in front of you.
Inhale; as you exhale stretch forward and attempt to reach your
toes. Do not force the motion. As you find it easier to do, stretch
progressively farther.

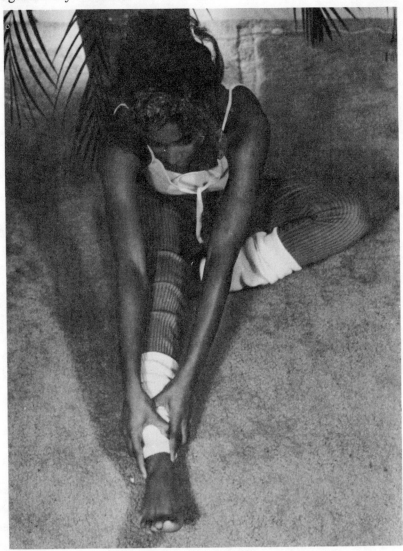

Touch your toes, but try not to force the motion.

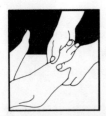

VARICOSE VEINS

Varicose veins constituted a serious nuisance as far back as Cleopatra's time. Now, one in seven Americans has this circulatory imbalance. (One in four women has it.) Varicosity, virtually unknown in nonindustrialized countries, is today one of the most common ailments of the circulatory system.

Veins are part of the body's maintenance department. They collect trash put out by the cells and haul it away. Veins also return blood from the body to the heart for recirculation. The legs' major veins are the longest in the body, running from the ankle up to the groin.

When flat feet, arthritic knees, or back ailments put too much pressure on veins, that combines with the adverse effects of gravity to dilate or stretch them. The veins may then become twisted or distorted, preventing the valves from directing the normal flow of venous blood from the leg. Varicose veins are the result. Pressure within the vein is greater in the lower part of the leg because this area bears the brunt of the body's weight.

In women the symptoms of varicose veins—burning or itching legs or a tired, weak feeling in the legs—can heighten during menstruation. But because they have an extra layer of fat under the skin, they hide varicose veins better than men.

HELP FOR VARICOSE VEINS

Massage, diet, and exercise are the most efficient ways to prevent varicose veins. The following are tips for everyday relief. (If the problem is severe, consult a physician before using any technique described.)

—Elevate your legs every chance you get. This takes the pressure off them and helps the leg pump rid itself of toxins.

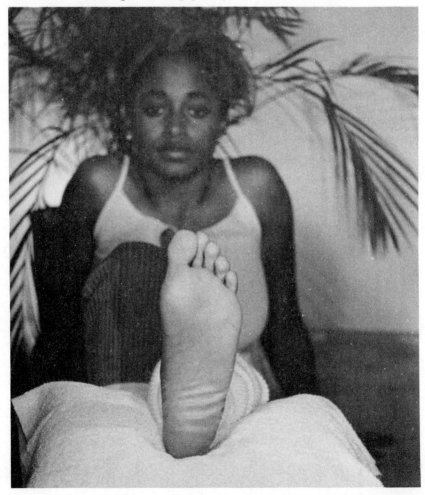

Elevate your legs as often as possible to relieve pressure on varicose veins.

—Follow a fat-reduction diet.

—Do not wear tight shoes, high heels, garters, or restricting socks that may hinder circulation.

—If you have the type of job that has you standing on your feet for long periods of time, walk around from time to time to stimulate circulation and distribute the pressure to different parts of the legs.

—Sleep with pillows under your feet.

Self technique: Stroking and compression in the area of the painful veins will always help. Place the center of a towel (twisted like a rope) under the sole of your foot. Press your foot into the towel while pulling the towel from left to right like a pulley. This balances the circulation in the lower leg.

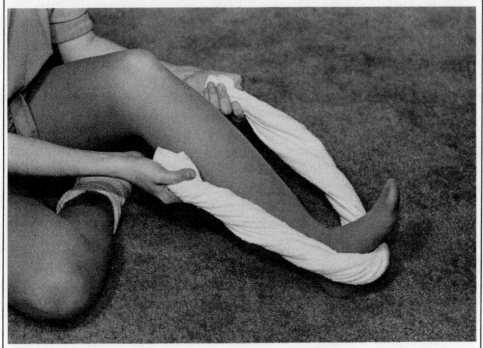

Using towel massage to balance circulation in the legs.

Exercise: Jogging (except on cement surfaces) and cycling strengthen the muscles and circulatory system in the legs as well as throughout the body.

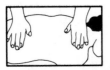

CELLULITE

Cellulite is composed of fat, lingering unmetabolized toxins, and wastes. It is often a problem because it simply refuses to go away. It remains after fat disappears, even after strenuous attempts at dieting and exercise, because it is enclosed in a gel-like substance below the skin surface. Cellulite attracts more water and toxins and eventually expands, leaving unsightly flab.

Some people try to burn waste fat through extreme diets or exercise programs, but while the body can burn off regular fat, more is needed to dissipate these unwanted pockets of gel-like fat.

Since the fatty tissue content in women is greater than in men, they are more prone to cellulite problems. In women's thighs and buttocks, fat is held in pouches of connective tissue arranged in a honeycomb-like pattern. As women age, the connective tissue shrinks and loses its elasticity. The skin overlying these areas contracts. If the fat cells under the skin do not shrink to match, dimpling or rippling appears on the surface of the skin. Because men have more connective tissue than women and because it exists in a crisscrossing pattern that better supports the skin, they experience less dimpling.

Among the causes of cellulite are: improper diet, including too many animal fats; lack of exercise; poor circulation; poor lymphatic drainage; tension.

Since all of these factors contribute to cellulite, all must be approached together for an effective treatment. (Birth control pills, hered-

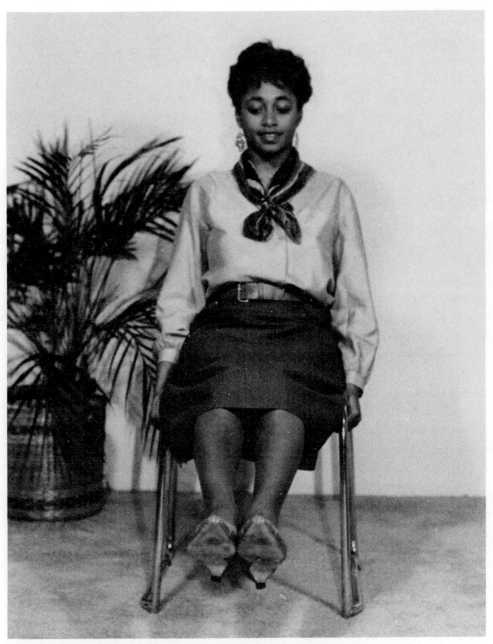

Leg lifts can reduce cellulite by toning the muscles.

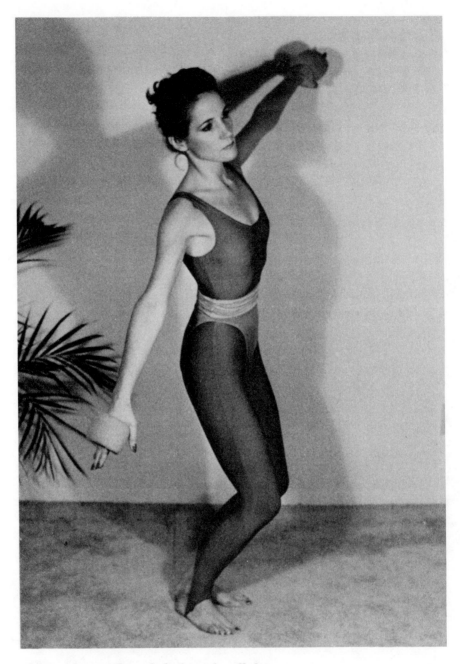

Lean from side to side to help banish cellulite.

itary factors, and pregnancy may also need to be considered.) Cellulite *can* be effectively prevented and in many cases diminished. Toxic wastes must be drained from fat areas through proper diet, a regular exercise program, and cleansing. Proper breathing should be learned as a means to reduce stress and tension. Finally, massage should be used to break up trapped substances and restore elasticity and tone to tissues.

Exercises:

1. Lying on the floor on your side, bring one leg up, then lower slowly. Repeat seven times with each leg. Turn on your other side and repeat with your other leg. Be sure that you move only your leg, so the pressure is on the thigh area.

2. Lie on your back. Bring the soles of your feet together, hold to a count of ten, then release slowly. Repeat this five times.

3. Lie on your back and make bicycling motions with your legs. Pedal with both legs.

4. With both arms to your sides, lean over at the waist to either side, as far as you comfortably can. Swing from one side to the other.

Self techniques:

1. Sitting on the floor, stretch one leg straight out in front of you, and put the foot of your other leg inside the knee of the outstretched leg. Grasp the muscle that will protrude on the inner thigh with your four fingers and thumb. Knead along the inner thigh.

2. For the outer thigh, stand upright and massage the muscle that protrudes along the outer part of the upper leg.

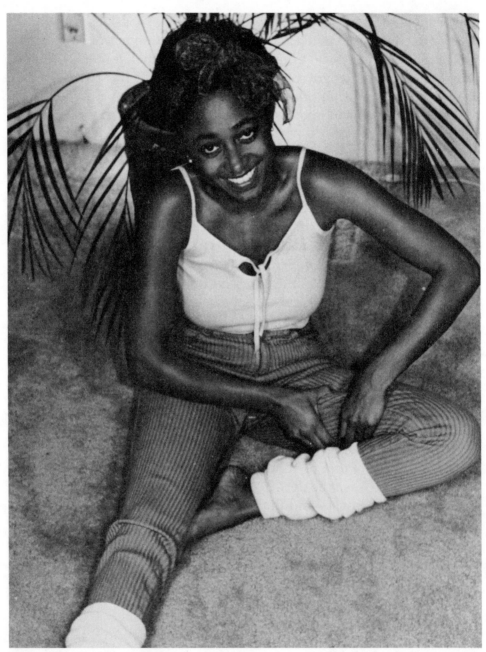

Massaging the inner thigh.

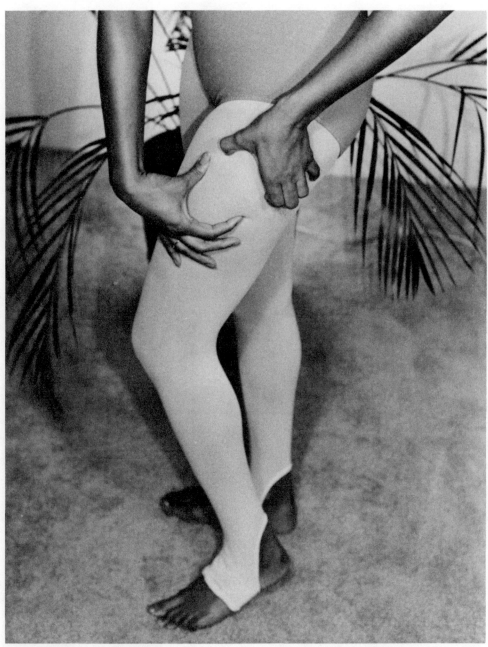

Massaging the outer thigh.

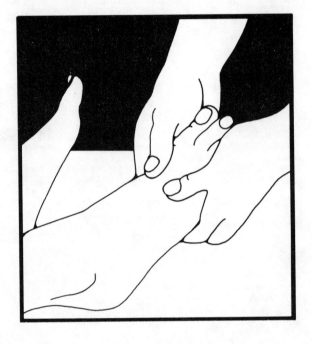

13
Best Foot Forward

Perhaps the most important and also the most vulnerable parts of our bodies are our feet. We use them constantly, since they provide support for the entire body. Feet that are tired or aching will cause an overall nagging ache or pain and can detract from beauty and good posture in every part of the body. When they are massaged and soothed, the feeling is deliciously refreshing.

Most of us neglect our feet, but they are beautiful when properly cared for—not merely what we get around on. In fact, the foot has been one of the most sensuous and pampered body parts for thousands of years. The Chinese considered it a sex symbol and favored a technique called foot binding for women, in which the heel bone is lifted into an almost vertical position, as if one were wearing high heels. The bound foot became a symbol of status as well as a fetish. In America, the foot was used by the early settlers for taking measurements. Numerous expressions have arisen involving the word *foot:* "best foot forward," "getting a foot in the door."

Each foot contains 26 bones with 33 joints, linked by more than

100 ligaments. Muscles, tendons, and ligaments keep it in different positions. There are a few common foot problems that are worth noting:

Fallen arches—Each normal foot has two important arches. One runs lengthwise from the heel to the ball of the foot. The second runs across the ball of the foot. These provide the spring needed for walking. In the condition known as flat feet, the arches have fallen so that the weight is borne on the sole of the foot as well as on the ball and heel.

Athlete's foot—This ringworm infection can be avoided by keeping the feet clean, dry, and cool. It is caused by bacteria, and first appears in the toe clefts. It may look like split or flaking pieces of dead white skin. For relief, give the feet as much air as possible, soak them, and massage away the dead skin. Wear clean white cotton socks with shoes. The health craze has more people using public health clubs, which poses a special hazard: Never walk on the wet floors barefooted!

Calluses are circumscribed areas of the skin thickened by hypertrophy or a layer of epidermis caused by friction or pressure. (After a fracture, a new growth of bony tissue surrounds bone ends as part of the reparative process.) Hardened skin offers protection for parts that suffer friction or pressure but may leave the area painful if rubbed against shoes or socks.

To prevent calluses, never wear shoes that are too tight. Soak feet in warm water and remove the callus by massaging with an emery board or pumice stone.

Corns are a type of callus whose corn-shaped core causes pain. They are usually caused by ill-fitting shoes. Removal should be left to a professional.

Bunions (hammertoes) are hard swellings at the base of the big toe. Ill-fitting shoes cause the big toe to bend in. Also, poor posture will place extra pressure on this area and encourage the formation of bunions.

Bone spurs are bony growths that develop on bones within the foot. They are made up of calcium, which is deposited by the body in response to increased pressure on a bone.

Heel fissures are painful cracks that form at the back or sides of the heel. They are sometimes associated with calluses. They are often found in overweight people and those who wear backless shoes.

For relief, soak the feet for 10 minutes a day in warm water and sea salt.

Develop a regular foot regime: After a bath or shower, massage the feet in olive oil, then cover with clean white cotton socks. Get in the habit of scrubbing the heels with a loofah. Lose weight if you are overweight.

Achilles tendon is a part of the foot that receives stress and overuse in many dancers and athletes. Because it is a sensitive area, it may be a source of weakness. Achilles tendonitis is an inflammation of the tendinous insertion of the calf muscle into the back of the calf heel. It causes pain in the posterior part of the heel and can extend upward to the calf. The condition is aggravated by the use of steroids; an excessive increase in activity level (e.g., running up hills, climbing, being *en pointe* in ballet); extreme changes in footwear (from high heels to flat shoes); and failure to properly stretch the tendon before exercise.

BASIC FOOT CARE

Wash feet at least once a day, soak in sea salt and warm water.

Dust feet to avoid friction and odor.

Cut toe nails straight across and not at edges. If left untrimmed or too long, they will look unattractive and also cause problems.

Wear clean hosiery.

Keep feet free of corns and calluses.

Wear comfortable shoes.

Remember that the feet reflect the body's total alignment, so be aware of how you exert pressure on them. Watch your posture.

Practice exercises that give the feet grace and balance.

Avoid tight garters and hosiery that may restrict the circulation.

A typical worker walks up to 7½ miles a day and a housewife walks up to 10 miles a day. In a lifetime the average person walks up to 70,000 miles. That is three times around the world. No wonder our feet hurt! Therefore the most important way to ensure beautiful, tension-free feet is to massage, massage, massage.

Self and esthetic techniques:

Stroking: This is a gentle, sensual technique that works best on the feet. Grasp the feet securely with both hands. Stroke both the top and bottom of the foot. You may want to apply oil to insure smooth strokes. Don't forget the tips of the toes. They are perhaps the most sensitive part of the foot, and are connected to the sinus reflex through the nervous system. This technique will help clear the sinuses.

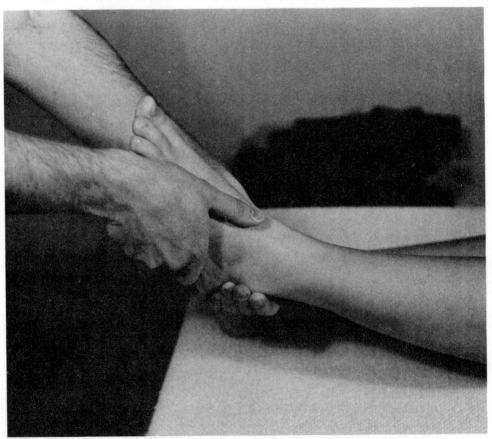

Stroking the foot, using long, gentle, but deep-rubbing motions. (A)

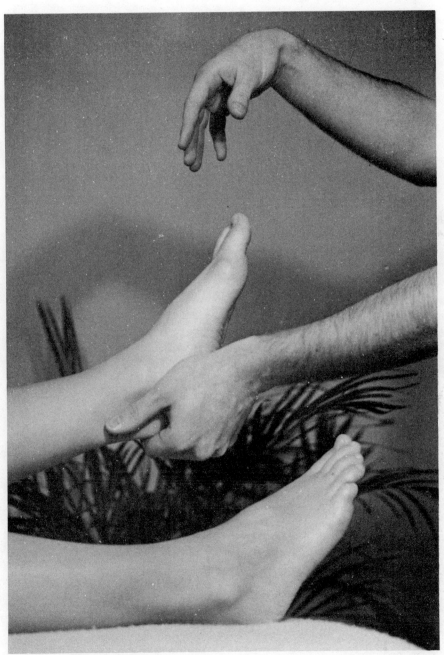

Stroking the foot. (B)

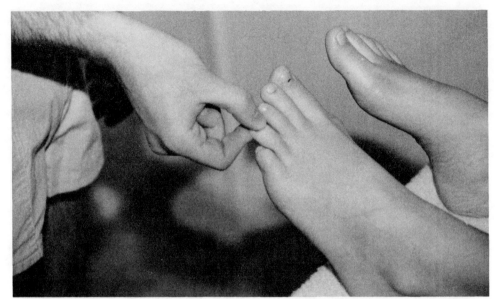

The tips of the toes are the most sensitive, sensual massage points in the feet.

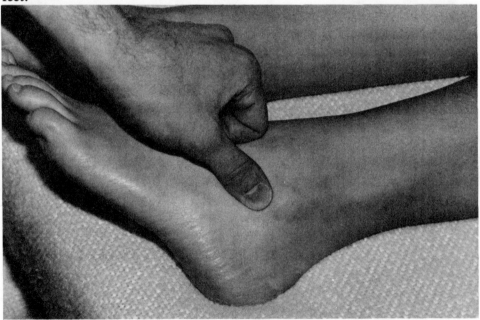

Massaging the foot's energy-giving pressure point.

Pressure point for increasing energy: Apply gentle pressure just below and outside of the ankle. To find it, close your eyes and slowly rotate your index finger in this area until you feel a small indentation, or feel a slight tingling sensation. Hold the pressure for a count of fifteen, then release. Repeat this three times.

All reflex points terminate in the foot, and the center of the foot connects to the entire reflex system. Apply gentle pressure and hold, then rotate the palm or the center of the finger in small motions, rubbing out tension.

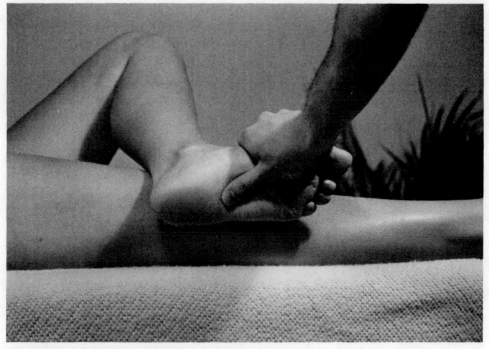

The center of the foot is a vital massage point.

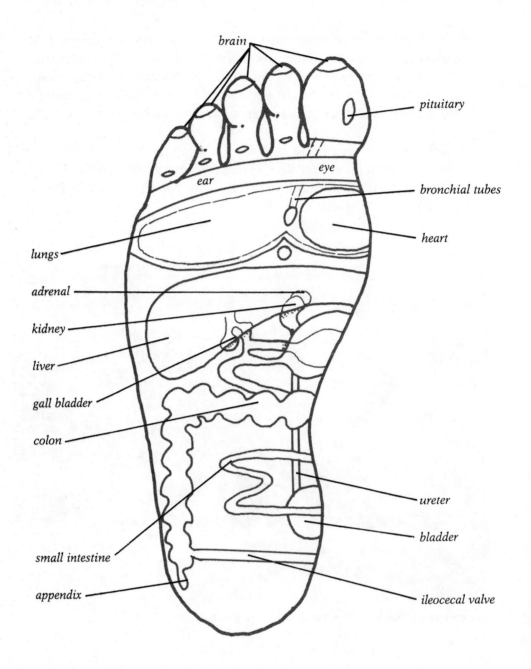

brain

pituitary

eye

ear

bronchial tubes

heart

lungs

adrenal

kidney

liver

gall bladder

colon

ureter

bladder

small intestine

appendix

ileocecal valve

Organ-related pressure points in the right and left foot.

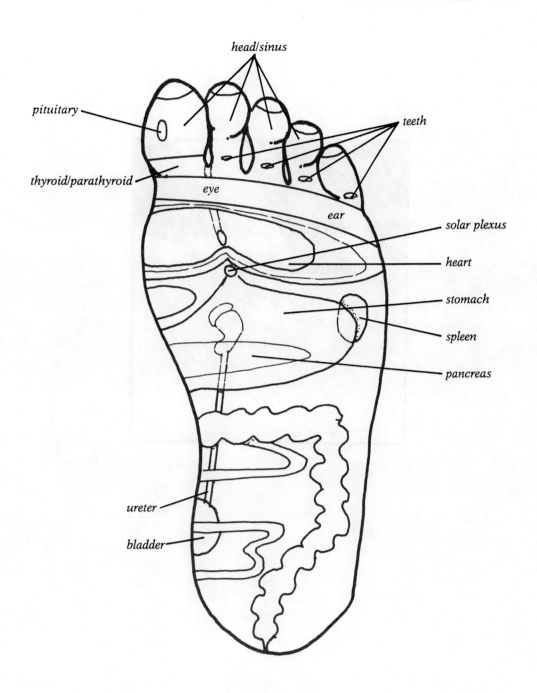

head/sinus

pituitary

teeth

thyroid/parathyroid

eye

ear

solar plexus

heart

stomach

spleen

pancreas

ureter

bladder

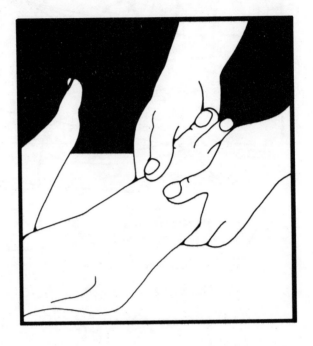

14
Do You Mind?

The mind is connected to the body. Our environment is directly reflected by our minds. All three are influenced by one another. The state of our physical health is associated with the state of social happiness, and our social activities can have an effect on our bodies.

Stress is a pressure exerted on something that causes a certain reaction. Stress is not necessarily either all good or all bad. Some stressful situations are integral to our achievements; they may stimulate our optimal efforts. A salesman who must reach a quota finds himself in a stressful situation. He reaches deep inside, makes calls he might not ordinarily make, gets out on the street, goes from store to store. By the end of the week, he has not only met his quota, but has been driven to reach a career high in sales.

As with the salesman, you will experience many stages of internal activity during stressful moments. Stress can make you run faster, jump higher, think faster, and accomplish feats that supercede your normal potential. Stress can be the cheerleader or booster squad that pushes you to new heights.

On the other hand, stress can also be the cause of both mental and physical upsets, and long-term stress can lead to difficulties beyond our control; it can wear us down. Harmful stress is intense exertion, strain, and effort; the wear and tear of everyday life. Yet it is not necessarily the amount of stress but how we choose to handle it that determines how it will affect us.

Visualize stress as a balloon. The balloon is empty at first. We begin filling it with air. If we fill it just right, the balloon will take its familiar shape and function as a balloon should. The stress of forcing air into the balloon has caused it to expand. (Remember, some stress is good.) However—that's right, you guessed it—when we keep pumping air into it, more air, more air, and more air . . . it explodes!

As it is with the balloon and too much air, so it can be with our bodies and too much pressure. So let's examine exactly how stress works.

Every one of us is under some degree of stress in today's fast-paced world. Pollution, noise, war, divorce, crime, rising costs—the quality of life appears to be changing. But rather than just complaining about the changing times, we have the task of adjusting to it.

There is a mechanism in the body called the fight-or-flight response. This is the first line of defense against stress. When the body is presented with a stressful situation, it is forced to react. Either it will meet the situation head-on or it may temporarily file it away for action at a later date, or dismiss it altogether. Keep in mind that the situation will never go away of its own accord. So doing the latter will eventually cause the problem to surface—maybe as a headache or "pain in the neck."

This first fight-or-flight reaction causes the adrenal glands to begin flowing. The hormones released by the adrenal glands must have vitamins A, B, C, and E or they will rob the body of its valuable supply. Stress has already begun to place extra demands on our sensitive bodies. Remember, each time we face a stressful situation, the body is being robbed of vital nutrients in its effort to meet or resist the problem.

Next, an entire series of psychological functions is called into play. Perspiration and respiration increase, body temperature rises, and speech quickens. Sound familiar? In other words, the body begins to move at double time.

Acids are also released in the stomach. These acids will soon burn a hole in the lining of the stomach tissue. The blood vessels in the shoulders, neck, and head constrict. Blood pressure rises and the heart rate increases. The heart works harder to push blood through the smaller arteries. When the blood vessels become too small, blood and oxygen do not reach the brain. Look out, here come the headaches. Muscles contract and become tight. We may clench our fists or grit our teeth— more tension.

Thus, all sorts of adverse reactions occur when we are under physical or emotional stress. The body affects the mind, and the mind affects the body.

There is also a price to be paid for not resisting stress at all, for simply denying its existence. Often, we will bury the truth and hide the stress in our bodies. This will undoubtedly manifest itself in some way as time goes on.

Negative emotions can detract from our health and happiness. Facing reality may not be the easiest thing to do, but it is certainly the healthiest. Learn to accept what you cannot change. Many of us get upset about circumstances that are beyond our control. This may lead to frustration, a harmful emotion. Frustration may cause premature aging and a host of other bodily ills.

Get away from it all from time to time. Clear your mind and see things for what they are. When you are confused, upset, or just plain out of it, take some personal time to restore yourself. Then approach the problem again; it will never seem as bad then. Look at both sides, especially the bright side of things. If you appear to be losing, learn from it. There is a valuable lesson in everything. By all means, avoid popping pills for everything that goes wrong in your life.

Don't be a worrywart. Using too much mental energy will wear you down. Talk out your problems. Often we take the attitude of being doomed to suffer alone. This usually leads to a lot of pent-up emotion that eventually shows on the outside. That's right . . . it's one cause of aging and wrinkling. And yes, it's true, you *can* actually worry until your hair starts to fall out!

Words have a power all their own. Some may present the body with

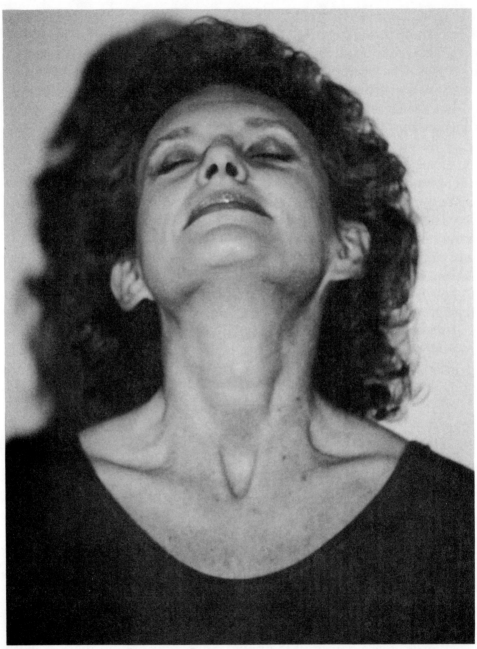

Relax and let stress pass out of you.

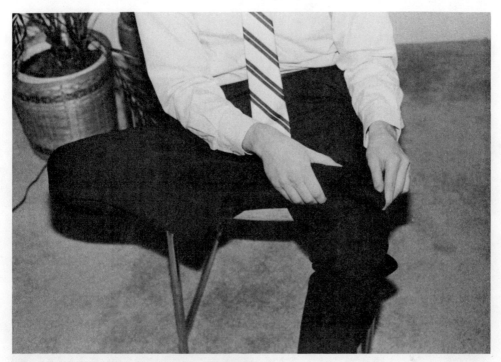

Time out for a foot massage in the office.

pictures of despair and depression, others with images of happiness, beauty, and pleasure. See the difference words can make:

"I hate my job." . . . "I am ready for a better job."

"It's a load on my chest." . . . "I have a lot to do."

"He's a pain in the neck." . . . "He and I can work it out."

Here are some negative words:

- hate
- no
- don't
- jealousy
- guilt
- war
- anger
- fear

Here are some positive words:

- love
- compassion
- forgiveness
- courage
- beauty
- happiness
- hope

Positive and negative emotions and actions are mentioned here because they do have an effect on our well-being. Each emotion has a particular effect on the body, which in turn affects the way we look and the way we feel.

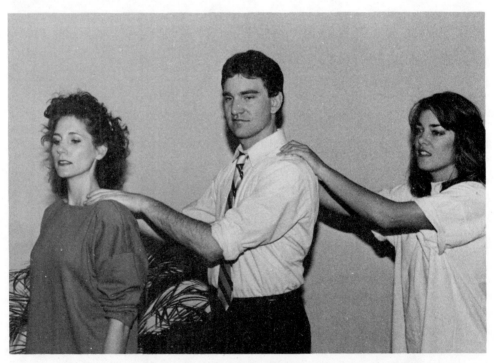

Passing energy and relieving each other's stress in the midst of daily pressures can be pleasurable and beneficial.

Here are some techniques to help us deal with stress:

- Try to plan ahead whenever possible.
- Use mental imagery to visualize a positive outcome of your activity.
- Get as much background as you can on the situation you are about to enter.
- Become aware of the advanced physical symptoms of stress:
  clenched fists or toes
  gritting of teeth or a tight jaw
  sweaty palms or forehead
  headache
  nervousness
  short, quick breaths
  fast, loud speech
  stomach "in a knot"
- Adopt an overall positive attitude.
- Speak up and stand up for your views.
- Always breathe, breathe, breathe!

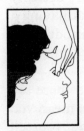

"HE WHO LAUGHS LAST, LAUGHS BEST . . ."

Think positively and your life *will* become more positive. This does not mean that miracles will fall from the sky, but it does mean that a change for the better will happen. Use daydreaming and mental fantasies as a way of releasing tension. It's okay to daydream—after all, fantasies are a part of the fun of life. Laughter can relieve stress and promote circulation. It will also increase skin tone.

Here are some facts about attitude and well-being to keep in mind:

- We are as happy in our lives as we decide to be.
- What is on your mind may affect the way you feel.
- It is impossible to have a good laugh and look sad at the same time.
- A warm smile will make you feel better.
- Laughter is a form of mental exercise; it can benefit the heart because the deep respiration that accompanies it can increase oxygen in the blood. It exercises the heart, thorax, stomach, chest, diaphragm, and lungs.
- Humor may stimulate the endocrine system, producing a substance called endorphine that affects the brain's pleasure center.

WHO'S ON YOUR MIND?

"No man is an island." No person stands alone. This does not, however, mean that your phone should be jumping off the hook all the time. In fact, many people who always wait for the phone to ring may actually lack a sense of security and self-assurance. They may feel that having a lot of friends is a sign of their popularity. This can be counterproductive, especially since they may find eventually that there is never time to be by themselves.

It is important to like and feel good about yourself, and there are many things you can do alone. Enjoying life does not always mean you have to be with someone else. Take the time to get to know yourself really well. It can be a lifetime job. It can also be rewarding.

Of course, a good relationship is a valuable thing to have. Sharing and caring can bring many positive benefits. Finally, whether it is with your child, your lover, or your best friend, remember to have plenty of FUN! FUN! FUN!

Index